CARING FOR CAREGIVERS

CRITICAL FILIPINX STUDIES

Robyn Magalit Rodriguez, editor

caring for caregivers

FILIPINA MIGRANT WORKERS
AND COMMUNITY BUILDING
DURING CRISIS

Valerie Francisco-Menchavez

University of Washington Press / *Seattle*

Caring for Caregivers was made possible in part by a grant from the Bulosan Center for Filipinx Studies at the University of California, Davis.

Copyright © 2024 by the University of Washington Press

Design by Ani Rucki

Composed in Minion Pro, typeface designed by Robert Slimbach

All rights reserved. No part of this publication may be reproduced or transmitted in any form or by any means, electronic or mechanical, including photocopy, recording, or any information storage or retrieval system, without permission in writing from the publisher.

Photographs by the author unless otherwise noted.

UNIVERSITY OF WASHINGTON PRESS

uwapress.uw.edu

Cataloging information is available from the Library of Congress.

LIBRARY OF CONGRESS CONTROL NUMBER: 2024945440

ISBN 9780295753133 (hardcover)
ISBN 9780295753140 (paperback)
ISBN 9780295753157 (ebook)

∞ This paper meets the requirements of ANSI/NISO z39.48-1992 (Permanence of Paper).

CONTENTS

Acknowledgments *vii*

Introduction *1*

CHAPTER 1 / No Work, No Pay *29*

CHAPTER 2 / Invisible Frontliners in the Time of Coronavirus *57*

CHAPTER 3 / Relationality as a Politics of Care *85*

CHAPTER 4 / Kuwentuhan and Intergenerational Activism *115*

Epilogue *147*

Notes *163*

Works Cited *175*

Index *195*

For Pila "Bill" Siukituatonga
For all the caregivers in my family
For all the caregivers

ACKNOWLEDGMENTS

This book's idea incubation, research, movement, and organization-building efforts, self-reflection, writing, revising, and finalizing took a decade. But in the final stretch of writing and revision, my family experienced a huge loss with the tragic death of my brother-in-love, Pila "Bill" Siukituatonga, beloved husband of my sister, Alexie Rae, and the father of their four children. Bill's light and love was the family he was building with Alexie. They had their first child, Kanoah Tasileki, in April 2014. In his new role as father, Bill looked forward to each milestone he discovered with Kanoah—crawling, walking, talking, first football or baseball game. He beamed seeing Kanoah's every little bit of growth. Bill and Alexie welcomed their daughter, Melana Reme, in August 2016. Thrilled about a baby girl, Bill and Alexie celebrated with bursts of pink and flowers. Melana was the apple of Bill's eye, his beautiful girl. Sadly, Melana passed away the following November, only three months old, from SIDS. With broken hearts, Bill and Lexie held each other close through this impossible time, holding on to Kanoah to remind them to live. After many months of heartbreak and healing, they welcomed their third child, Ezekiel Viliami, or Ziggy to all of us, in June 2018. With their new bundle of joy in hand, Bill and Alexie looked forward to raising brothers in Raiders gear and with a love of all things Disney. They took both boys to Disneyland multiple times a year, falling in love with their beautiful sons and giving them the Disney magic over and again, even between park visits. In December 2021, Rico Kingston, their fourth child, came into the world. A sweet, mild-mannered baby boy, Rico had to have cranial surgery right after his first birthday, in 2023. Only six months later, in July 2023, Bill would transition into one of our family's spirit guides.

Bill was and continues to be such a significant part of our lives. My husband, Raul, and Bill were fast friends and as thick as thieves. Raul's and my children, Aya and Cy, considered Bill a second dad, calling him Teti, the Tongan word for Dad. For me, Bill's unrelenting support for all the things I do—getting my PhD, writing books, raising kids, running miles, lifting weights—became the bedrock for how far and high I reached. Both Bill and Alexie were, and always are, my biggest supporters, even if they didn't quite know exactly what the next steps were. They just both believed in me. They were both only too happy to cheer me on when I got to the finishing lines. To this day and in all my days, I carry so much gratitude in my heart for knowing and loving Bill as my brother. After he passed away, I almost gave up, convincing myself I couldn't finish this book. It was Alexie who reminded me that Bill would want me to keep living, keep reaching, keep making goals and achieving them. Thank you, Bill, for loving my sister, your kids, my parents, my children, my husband and me, so fiercely. Bill, we are trying every day to honor you in song and story, in life and living, in prayer and love. We miss you so much. We all hope we are making you proud.

This book could not have been possible without the Filipina and Filipino caregivers who lent me their stories and experiences. I am grateful for all the caregivers who participated in interviews, surveys, and *kuwentuhan* in the many phases of this research. My thanks to the many grassroots and community-based organizations who collaborated with me to create and conduct research that sought to serve the needs of Filipino migrant workers. Thank you to the Filipino Community Center in San Francisco and the Pilipino Association of Workers and Immigrants (PAWIS) in the South Bay Area, the organizations that anchored the research projects I helped to conduct in 2011 and 2020, respectively. The leaders in these organizations are many, but I would especially like to recognize Mario de Mira, Tina Shauf-Bajar, Rowena Cayetano, Tetet Naval, Angelica Cabande, Lyra Ibarra-Samson, Faye Lacanilao, Michael Luat, Ryan Leano, Joel Zabanal, Edwin Herrera, and Bernadette Herrera, who volunteered and ran the Workers' Rights Program at the Filipino Community Center in the first version of the CARE Project. In PAWIS, I'd like to thank Felwina Opiso-Mondina, Rolly Mondina, Tess Brillante, Aleth Brown for their generous collaboration and consultation on conducting kuwentuhan during COVID-19. I am thankful for grassroots and National Democratic organizations in the Bay Area, GABRIELA, League of Filipino Students, and Anakbayan, that helped to bring these projects to life with their critical analysis and organizational and logistical support. In 2011, Pia Cortez, Charm Consolacion, Princess Bustos, Melissa Reyes, Ivy Climacosa, Sandra Panopio, and Alexis David were GABRIELA SF members who were key in facilitating the kuwentuhan sessions, data analysis, and caring for the caregiver co-researchers. I'm thankful to campus-based Filipino student organizations such as the Pilipino American Collegiate Endeavor at San Francisco State University and Kasamahan at the University of San Francisco, whose members in 2011, Caroline Calderon, Sunshine Roque, Allen Ocampo, and Evelyn Obamos, were crucial to running the research programs with the Filipino Community Center. More recently, I am grateful for the activism and political organizing of the California Domestic Worker Coalition, especially Megan Whelan and Tina Shauf-Bajar, and Gabriela Oakland with my *kasamas* Sam Sipin, Alisa de los Reyes, Claire Valderrama-Wallace, and Elaine Kathryn Andres, who have followed up with me and welcomed my family into our organizing activities. My participation in these progressive organizing spaces has helped me to frame the ideas in the book and the praxis I carry out in my daily life.

My former undergraduate and graduate students at SF State have been essential collaborators, thought partners, and co-researchers. I list them here knowing that this small recognition in these pages cannot account for their brilliant contributions to this intellectual project and my growth as a professor, scholar, educator, and activist. These amazing social scientists partnered with me on tasks like recruiting their own family members for survey and kuwentuhan collection, transcription, data analysis, writing, presenting and publication, organizing and advocacy for Filipino caregivers. Thank you to Kristal Osorio, Tim Mendoza, La Raine Gonzales, Alyssa Barquin, Tanya Yared, Knoble Tankiamco, Lawrence Rirao, Samir Shrestha, Aaron Alejo, Jesus Alvarez, and Kay Buban. Undergraduate and graduate students from other universities also joined my research groups, and I'm grateful for their time and commitment: Edwin Carlos, Elaika Celemen, Renee Zapata, and Chloe Punsalan.

Many colleagues and peers, and their brilliant work, have been vital resources for the development of this manuscript. I'm grateful to Robyn Rodriguez for her patient and constant presence and collaboration in this project, and so many other visions, dreams, and initiatives. As an intellectual and political conspirator, Robyn has helped me tell the stories of caregivers and strategize on how to use many platforms to elevate the basis for solidarity with migrant workers for years. Through wins and grief, Robyn has been an example to me for creating intentional relationships that center on care and love. Through her work in the historic Bulosan Center for Filipinx Studies at the University of California, Davis, which has transformed into the Amado Khaya Initiative, I have been able to present my work and strike up collaborations with doctoral students and scholars.

I want to acknowledge James McMaster, who was at the University of Wisconsin, Madison, and is now at George Washington University and invited me to the Relations of Care Across and After Worlds virtual conference in May 2021 to share a keynote about Filipino caregiver organizing, an early version of chapter 3. After this conference, I coauthored an article with Katherine Nasol published in *American Behavioral Scientist* on the concepts of dual crises in the caregiving industry that informed the framing of chapter 3. In the summer of 2021, I was a participant in the Imagining America, Stories of Change program led by Erica Kohl and Christina Preston; this came at a crucial time to help me flesh out the details of chapter 2 in a multimedia collaborative project with PAWIS. Through this work, some concepts in chapter 2 were developed in an article published in *Alon: Journal for Filipinx American and Diasporic Studies* coauthored with Kristal Osorio and Elaika Celemen. In the summer of 2022, I was awarded a Fulbright to Cebu, Philippines, and was able to moonlight as a visiting scholar at the Asian Research Institute at Yale-National University of Singapore, where Brenda Yeoh, Theodora Lam, and Chand Somaiah welcomed my ideas and work. I am grateful to the three of them. I am also thankful to Ilyan Ferrer and Conely de Leon, Filipino Canadian scholars who kindly invited me to collaborate on their Social Sciences and Humanities Research Council grant project on multidirectional immigration, aging, and care. The years-long collaboration with Ilyan, Conely, and Robyn helped shape my ideas on chapters 1 and 5, culminating with a retreat and virtual presentation in May 2023. I'd like to thank Jocelyn Olcott and Tania Rispoli at the Revaluing Care in the Global Economy collaborative at Duke University, who hosted a close reading and discussion of chapter 4 in October 2023 wherein Anju Paul and Pallavi Banerjee gave me generous comments that helped with my revisions. I am thankful for the following academic organizations—Association for Asian American Studies, National Women's Studies Association, and American Sociological Association—as spaces for presentation and dialogue with scholars on earlier versions of this manuscript.

My ability to braid together my scholarship and research with teaching and mentoring at SF State is made possible by my understanding and passionate colleagues at the Department of Sociology and Sexuality Studies. I count myself lucky to work at a university where I can create and nourish meaningful collegial relationships with my colleagues across disciplines, departments, and colleges who have invited me to give lectures, sit in writing groups, and create impactful change at our institution. I thank Angi Fillingim, Ikaika Gleisberg, Jen Reck, Clare Sears, Sherria Taylor, David Rebanal, Supriya Misra, Zubaida Qamar, Cesar Che Rodriguez, Nicole Bolter, Aiko Yoshino, Autumn Thoyre, Carina Gallo, Arlene Daus-Magbual, Allyson Tintiangco-Cubales, Grace Yoo, Fatima Alaoui, Laura Mamo, Emiko Takagi, Savi Malik, and Marty Martinson. Scholars who have modeled a path of authenticity and a prioritization of health outside of SF State also have my thanks: Subini Annamma, Grace Chang, Celine Parreñas Shimizu, Dawn Lee, and OiYan Poon.

Critical Filipinx Studies is my homeplace, as bell hooks has coined referencing site(s) of resistance and groups of people where one can restore ourselves. In different formulations of Critical Filipinx Studies scholars and community, I have recovered all parts of myself as Filipina, woman, mother, partner, daughter, sister, activist, scholar, educator, and author. I am indebted to Filipinx American and diasporic and Philippine scholars for their unrelenting encouragement and constructive criticism of my praxis. The Critical Filipinx Studies Collective, of which I am part, has provided a space for me, and others, to be true to our scholar-activist leaning while providing necessary camaraderie as we journey through academia. From early book proposal drafts to virtual writing sessions, these brilliant people have been pillars in my work, and for that I am appreciative to Mike Viola, Lorenzo Perillo, Joy Sales, Tracy Buenavista, Amanda Solomon Amorao, Jan Padios, Josen Diaz, Lucy Burns, Melissa-Ann Nievera-Lozano, Wayne Jopanda, Mike Castaneda, Sherwin Mendoza, Jason Magabo Perez, Miguel Abad, Mike Atienza, Rick Bonus, Martin Manalansan, Allen Punzalan Isaac, Sarah Raymundo, Yasmin Ortega, and Leny Ocasiones. A special note of gratitude for Faith Kares, a kindred spirit, who has taken care of me and my ideas in many ways through many years, a sisterhood that has helped me restore my faith in myself. In this network of Filipinx diasporic scholars, where I have intellectual partners in thinking about care work and Filipino migrants, I thank Dale Maglalang for early support on my quantitative analysis for the survey I launched in 2017. I also thank Katherine Nasol, Ethel Tungohan, Conely De Leon, Ilyan Ferrer, and Earvin Cabalquinto for being stalwart Filipinx diasporic scholars who have centered care work in their scholarship and created spaces for me to think and write and flourish alongside them. I want to acknowledge the master's and doctoral students I have the privilege of working and exchanging ideas with: Nelle Garcia, Jackie Stol, Veronica Salcedo, and Karen Villa. This group of people have expanded my notions of "mentorship," which is often too proprietary and damaging in the academy. With this growing set of Filipinx diasporic scholars, many not named here, I have cultivated my capacity to start and complete this work, and more important, to show up for other scholars in the field of Critical Filipinx Studies.

This book could not have come together without my amazing developmental editor, Jordan Beltran Gonzales, whose attention to detail and the big picture allowed me to meander into writing that had no direction and then revise my work toward coherency. I am grateful to Mike Baccam at the University of Washington Press, and the staff there, for believing in this book and giving me the opportunity to be the inaugural author in the book series for Critical Filipinx Studies with the University of Washington Press. The book's cover illustration is by the late Filipina artist Pacita Abad, whose *I Thought the Streets Were Paved with Gold* is an homage to the labor of immigrants: caregivers, domestic workers, construction workers, street vendors, and nurses. I am grateful for Pacita Abad and her ability to evoke our imagination and solidarity through art, something I aspire to in my writing.

An integral part of writing this book was planning for focused time to think, read, and write on repeat. For a mother of two young children, it took a village to create the gift of time for me. I thank my kasama-mamas and the *ninangs* of my children, Irma and Tina Shauf-Bajar, Rocky Rivera, Alexis David, Joanna Robledo-Maderazo, Jaynee Ruiz, and Jessica Cruz. I want to acknowledge my family's communities of care, the families of Josie and Mario de Mira, Rocky Rivera and Bambu, Abigail and David Mesa, Justine and Ben Pelina-Chan, Lorraine and Tai Yamaguchi, Roanna and Adam Nishimoto, Jamel and Doug Ponciano, Karmela and Ben Herrera-Billones, Ailed and Zach Swan-Paningbatan, Karlen and Jay Paningbatan, Michelle and Jay Pagsanjan, and Connie Huang.

My family of origin, whose stories are bound up in mine, have been my anchors in telling and living the story that is the through line to this book. Almost all of the first-generation immigrants in my parents' and grandparents' generations worked as caregivers in the United States. Underemployed and underpaid, many of them raised my 1.5 generation of siblings and cousins on meager salaries and worked to gain stable livelihoods through caregiving. I want to thank my maternal and paternal grandparents, Purificacion Viray Alcantara and Benito Alcantara and Remedios Luna Francisco and Porfirio Francisco for their humility and hard work as caregivers, supporting so many of our extended family, in the United States and in the Philippines. Priscilla Tolentino, the grandmother I grew up with, has been a source of inspiration and strength, always my biggest cheerleader in my academic journey. Thank you, Lola Prescy, for your unwavering support.

My husband's family of origin, the Menchavez family, has been a source of encouragement and logistical detail about Filipino American history about their lived experience in the East Bay Area from the late 1970s to the 1990s. The anchor to the Menchavez family migrations was an ebullient man named Godofredo Manuel, who passed away in November 2023. He and his wife, Joan Manuel, held down a gateway home in Daly City for many family members to land from Cebu, Philippines, into a life in the Bay Area. My in-laws, Jim and Amy Menchavez, have been storytellers and repositories of their family's oral history. They have been reliable care takers, not only for my kids but also for me during the writing process for this book. I am grateful for the many times they took Aya and Cy to the park while I wrote at a coffee shop nearby and when they allowed me to work on drafts of this book in their ancestral home in Cebu. I want to acknowledge Lolita and Domen "Pops" Duran, Rich and Tricia Menchavez, and Jocelyn and Rodney Pierre-Antoine for always affirming me in my journey as a mama scholar. I thank the many members of the Menchavez family from the Bay Area to Cebu.

To my Mama Irma and Papa Vernon Francisco, thank you for instilling in me the importance of faith, resilience, and love for family. Your sacrifices for our family to live and thrive here in the Bay Area are unfathomable, and I know this life has not always been kind, but you have in turn shown us, your children and now grandchildren, the kindness that was withheld from you. For this, we are indebted. To my Kuya Arve, thank you for taking responsibility for Lexie and me at such a young age, growing up way before it was time but always showing us that you love us. To my sister and best friend, Alexie Rae, it is one of the greatest gifts to be your sister. For all that you have endured, for all the strength you exude, for all the love you still have left, I thank you.

To my children, Aya Gabriela and Cy Andres, you have changed me. From my physical cells to my visions for the future, my life and my work has fire and ice because you two have given me the tremendous privilege of becoming your mother. Thank you for your gentle forgiveness for my many mistakes, for your unrelenting belief in the world that Papa and I continue to build for you, from pillow forts to playground missions, chores and the rules for bath and bedtime, chanting in marches and loving the communities we sustain. Aya, you are a firebrand. Your confidence and understanding will take you far; remember to take it easy sometimes. This world needs your fire and your softness. Cy, my loving boy, I follow your lead in feeling fully with your heart and big emotions, your curiosity and willingness to challenge yourself and, in turn, this world. I learn from you every day about what it is to be brave and to be so, so chill; please know we will always love you in all of your enthusiasm and unique talents. As the mother to both of you children, I have experienced your care for me and Papa. You have taught us that while we put in the kind of labor grown-ups contribute to make our family possible, your care work, for us, is just as essential. At the publication of this book, Aya is nine and Cy is seven; both must be credited as my crucial parts of developing this book as they have had a say in nearly every stage of this book.

Lastly, this book would not be possible without my love, Raul Francisco-Menchavez. Quite literally, Raul has been my most consistent intellectual sounding board for the ideas and theories I have formed in this book. In long car rides with napping children in the backseat, I have pitched outlines of chapters and the arc of this book to Raul. His feedback and questions, always sincere and necessarily nonacademic, helped me to stretch my abstractions into intuitive and grounding consequences for our families, communities, and society at large. When it was time for me to write, Raul held down family logistics, handed me plates of food and cups of water to nourish me, fixed my Zoom issues, mined his own family's archives, and drove me and our children to nature when this book felt too dense. Raul, in the two decades we have been in each other's lives, you have made so many of my dreams come true—in no fantastical way either. I dreamed up a degree, a home, a family, a book project, and together we have actualized all these things. Even in our lowest lows, you have created space for our family to mourn and to come back to love. Always back to love. Thank you, Raul, for always believing in me—and believing in us.

CARING FOR CAREGIVERS

INTRODUCTION

When my family immigrated from the Philippines to the United States in 1992, our first home was a care home in the San Francisco Bay Area. There, my paternal grandparents worked and took care of six elderly people. Even though my grandparents were both secondary school teachers in the fields of math and art in the Philippines, when they came to the United States through a petition from a relative, the work that was easiest to find was in long-term care. The living arrangement that my grandparents negotiated with their Filipino employer, the owner of the care home, was that my mother and my two siblings would share one room with my grandparents. Although this arrangement was not up to the licensing code, we were allowed to stay at the care home just until my mother got on her feet.

As many immigrants do, my family was trying to adapt to new conditions in the United States. My mother endeavored to find stable employment after leaving a decade-long practice as an established dentist in the Philippines and accruing debt to finance our migration. Through the friends she had in the Bay Area, she found work as a one-on-one caregiver in a city across the Bay. She shuffled back and forth from one Bay Area city to another, working and living with her charge—an elderly Filipina woman and her patient's family—on the weekdays and then coming back to us at the nursing home every weekend, where she helped my grandparents in their responsibilities as the main caregivers. On top of all of that, my mother was continually studying for the dental board exams here in the United States, saving up her wages for the exams and to support her children. Because the financial constraint for our newcomer lives necessitated immediate and stable work for the adults in my family, the living conditions for all of us revolved around the work of caregiving in the care home. If it meant we shared a cramped room as our sleeping quarters, or that we all pitched in to help with the daily tasks of running the care home, so be it, even if we didn't see our mother daily. Since my father had been left behind in the Philippines because of visa issues, we did not have another adult to help out, so we immigrant children were recruited into the family business—caregiving. Even as children, we knew that we had to help as much as we could.

Only a few years after my family arrived, my paternal grandmother passed away. And because the care home she worked at required new workers, my maternal grandparents took the jobs as caregivers. When the chain migration for my relatives brought uncles and aunts to the Bay Area, they too tapped into our church community and friends of friends to secure jobs as caregivers in different cities. Finally, when my father was able to join us in the United States, he overstayed his tourist visa, and without legal papers the only type of work he could find and keep was as a caregiver. As I grew into young adulthood, most of my family members worked as caregivers—my maternal and paternal grandparents, two uncles, four aunts, and my sister worked in the caregiving industry at some point. I share these pieces of my autobiography to locate myself not just as a scholar and researcher of Filipino caregivers but also as someone whose epistemological foundation is rooted in the history of Filipino immigrants who have worked in the caregiving industry. My position as an insider to this community allows me to extend the analysis in this book to include my own experiences growing up and working in a care home alongside my relatives. My outsider status as a scholar and professor gives me the space and opportunity to apply sociological analysis to the very complicated nature and conditions of caregiving.

Today when I field questions from media outlets about my research on the lives of Filipino caregivers, especially on stories about caregivers who experience tremendous abuse and exploitation in their jobs, I am asked, "Why are there so many Filipinos working as caregivers? Why do they stay as caregivers given that it is such hard work?" I have often wondered the same thing and about the closest people in my life who work as caregivers, my family. This book is an effort to understand that labor pattern for Filipino migrants—to explore the question of how and why they come to be caregivers for the aging population in this country. While I provide historical and systemic analysis on the ethnic economic niche of caregiving for Filipinos in the States, I also grapple with the microsociological aspects of the job and how they shape the lives of caregivers. I provide a close and intimate look at the level of skill, patience, and rigorous labor required of caregivers, despite their being considered low-skilled and low-waged. I present this dialectic dance between structural patterns of labor migration and care crisis and the daily experiences and concerns of caregivers to highlight that this industry is at once failing and a site for resistance and change.

I build on extant literature reporting on the arduous work conditions of formal Filipino caregivers.[1] I expand the understanding of precarity in caregiving work by examining the consequences and motivations Filipino migrants use to persist in this occupation. I draw from psychosocial frameworks to examine mental and physical health from the perspective of caregivers and explore the types of health outcomes, such as stress and fatigue, as a product of their strenuous labor conditions.[2] I balance the hyperlocal conditions of caregiving with the transnational sociocultural contexts that inform how and why caregivers make the decisions they do about their work.[3] Different from past studies of formal caregivers, I am committed to including the sociocultural and transnational contexts that inform Filipino migrants' decisions to continue working as caregivers under, at times, dangerous conditions because it is so imbricated in their day-to-day reasonings.

Instead of a book solely examining the conditions and organization of the caregiving industry in the United States, this book takes the holistic identities of Filipino caregivers as precarious workers, migrants, and transnational family members as social aspects that necessarily shape their experiences. I consider how Filipino caregivers leverage their transnational commitments to enact daily decisions in the workplace, as well as how they build a life where their feet are, in the United States, and where their hearts are, with their families in the Philippines. In these ways, this book contributes to the field of critical Filipinx American studies that insist on Filipinos' transnational lives as a key feature of their lives before their arrival and during their social incorporation to their new environs.

Race and racism are an inextricable fact from the history and contemporary stories of Filipino labor migrants. Cedric Robinson proposes that "racial capitalism" accrues exponential profit from the racialized and gendered labor assigned as less valuable and more disposable by white elites.[4] This theoretical frame does not avoid the complex and necessary ways in which race, ethnicity, gender, and sexuality contribute to capital accumulation, which is inextricable to political and economic power. In many ways, racial capitalism has long undergirded the paired dynamics of American imperial presence in the Philippines and settler colonial regimes in the United States producing sectors of racialized disposable workers for over a century.[5] Filipinos have historically figured into the American racial hierarchy of workers—from *sakadas*, or farmworkers, in Hawai'i, to agricultural workers in the Central Valley of California, to nurses in major American cities.[6] American immigration policies shape the streams of Philippine labor migration that deliver Filipinos to American domestic industries in need of workers in nursing, long-term care, early childhood care, and primary school teaching. Scholars have insisted that the stratification of low-wage domestic work reserved for immigrant women of color and women of color writ large is bolstered by state policies that refuse to allow for basic labor rights to this sector of workers.[7] In her recent dissertation, Dr. Katherine Nasol writes at length about this dynamic through what she calls a "neoliberal governance of care," which she defines as "an unequal allocation of care and reproductive labor across race, gender, and citizenship." Nasol argues that the neoliberal governing of care in the United States is enacted through anti-worker and anti-immigrant policies operating on dispossession of standard rights to health and safety in unregulated industries such as long-term care. Additionally, while care workers are essential to the American economy, neoliberal abandonment of social services that might provide assistance to many Filipino care workers leave them vulnerable to the industry's lack of protections.[8] To this end, I argue that the decades-long pattern of Filipino migration and incorporation into the long-term care industry as caregivers is a product of racial capitalism and a neoliberal governance of care. It is worth noting that care work in the United States also produces an uneven privilege on the basis of race, class, and gender as white and middle-class people are able to accumulate wealth while outsourcing domestic labor in their households. The transnational and domestic scale of the neoliberal governance of care has its sights on exponential profits from racialized and gendered immigrant care workers during a time when there is a critical need for care in an aging American population and especially as we live in times of a global epidemic.

I have always been interested in the paradoxical nature of care being both devalued yet deemed indispensable. The COVID-19 pandemic was and is a portal into which whole communities, cities, and nations began to reckon with the critical necessity of care and care workers. Hence, the analysis I present is a rumination on the significance of caregiving in the United States and how policies, or the lack thereof, continue to deleteriously shape the work and lives of caregivers. The current conditions of care and caregiving compels me to examine and theorize about the state of care work in this country. To do this, I center on the experiences of Filipino caregivers with the hope that they can shine a light on the gaping holes left behind by neoliberal states, like the United States, when care becomes at once a necessity and abandoned.

FILIPINO MIGRANTS AND THE CRISIS IN ELDERCARE

For more than a decade I have centered my research and political organizing on Filipino migrants working as caregivers to the elderly and as direct support care staff to developmentally disabled and chronically ill people. In that time there have been a few questions that have become routinely asked of me when I share my findings with the Filipino community in the United States, including various print, video, and social media outlets, academic conferences, students in classrooms, and, really, anyone who is trying to understand the plight of Filipino caregivers. Such questions guide this section. I review academic scholarship to explain the contemporary contexts of Filipino caregivers. I introduce theoretical frameworks that will help me analyze the complex nature of the labor required in caregiving and its impacts on various interpretations of care in the lives of Filipino migrants.

However, even as I try to tell this story in a linear fashion, the reality is that there are many parts of explaining the Filipino caregiver community that are circular, multilinear, and simultaneous with other Asian American migrations and elucidate the political and economic shifts in both the United States and the Philippines. Still, some historical contexts and theoretical frameworks situate the lives of so many Filipinos in the caregiving industry.

What Is a Caregiver and Where Do They Work?

As the Baby Boomer generation (people born between 1946 and 1964) continues to need specialized care in their post-retirement years, the US care crisis balloons. Arguably, the decline of the welfare state in the latter half of the twentieth century has resulted in the demand for caregivers for the elderly being at an all-time high.[9] Many ethnic immigrant women, with a formidable population of Filipina/o migrant caregivers, have answered the call as "formal care workers" in long-term care facilities.[10] Formal care workers, or "caregivers" as I refer to them in this book, are defined by the fact that they are paid for their work, as opposed to "informal caregivers," who are not paid to provide care to an individual or a group of individuals. Although some labor scholars and feminists insist on using the term "caregiver," "home health worker," or "worker," more broadly, to emphasize caring as labor, I invoke the term "caregiver" in this book, as many Filipino migrants refer to themselves as such and place great importance on their role as providing care. I use the terms "caregiver" and "care worker" interchangeably, the latter to refer to a wider range of care support workers.

Some of the participants in the research for this book identified themselves as "direct support care workers" or "direct care workers," the technical term for someone who is supporting with the daily living activities, health, and human services of an individual. "Personal care assistants" or "personal care attendants" are another category of care workers who assist with daily living activities but also attend to domestic work of cleaning, cooking, and maintenance of a home. All of these roles can be distinguished from other care workers who have medical training and responsibilities for in-home care after hospital stays or attending to chronic illnesses or disabilities. Certified nurse assistants and home health aides have at least seventy-five hours of training, have been conferred a license, and are under more regulation for their work than their unlicensed counterparts. Often caregivers are not required to have licenses and medical training, although many Filipino migrants included in this study actually had extensive experience in the medical field as nurses and medical staff before they came to the United States. Any collection of these care workers could be working at residential care facilities for the elderly in shifts, but most caregivers whose experiences are included in this book were unlicensed care workers.

Employment arrangements vary for caregivers. A caregiver could be employed by an individual or a family to care for a relative, whom I will refer to as "consumers" or "recipients" of care in order to emphasize recipients' choice and participation in the increased marketization of care.[11] Although consumers of care services are clearly making decisions about who and how to employ, when caregivers are employed by individuals or their families, the formal labor standards can fall to the wayside. Contracts, workers' compensation, sick leave, and paid time off are seldom involved in the hiring of a caregiver, as families do not consider themselves as "formal" employers of a caregiver; rather, families are paying someone "to help" with their needs. Employing a caregiver through individual arrangements are often sought through word of mouth by consumers and their families, although caregivers can also receive notice of opportunities through immigrant social networks. Securing work through Filipino relatives or friends becomes an important tether to the kinds of obligations caregivers feel as they navigate whether to stay in a job or not.

A second avenue by which caregivers in this study were employed was through agencies, some of which are for-profit or private while others are either contracted by state governments to provide care for consumers with Medicaid or referred by hospital systems. For example, California's In-Home Support Services is a consumer-directed program wherein individuals and clients can hire and fire caregivers and supervise the care of their relative while the state authorizes payment. Other for-profit agencies provide private clients with the care staff they might need for individual care or facilities' needs. While agencies can offer some of the standard worker benefits, such as contracts, taxes and deductions, workers' compensation, and health insurance, the companies are often looking to make profit from the caregivers they employ. A private client might pay what seems to be a livable hourly wage to their caregiver, but direct wages to the caregivers often suffer. Lastly, caregivers working with an agency often work multiple part-time jobs, as agencies can direct and redirect caregivers from one client to another.

Another avenue of employment for caregivers is work in larger care facilities, those with six beds or more. The lack of a federally funded system to provide long-term care for the aging population in countries like the United States and Canada has ushered in the growth of for-profit long-term residential care facilities.[12] After the 1965 passage of the Medicare and Medicaid programs in the United States, which pay for only short-term care for the aged and disabled, privatized nursing homes for long-term care increased parallel with the increasing needs of aging Americans.[13] In these settings, I use the terms "patients" and "clients" interchangeably as care workers' responsibility for limited medical assistance or assistance for daily living activities, respectively, describe the type of care work they engage in.

Historically, the privatization of the eldercare industry in the United States was a neoliberal response to the inability of the US government to provide ample government spending toward caring for a swelling aging population. It follows that the rapid expansion of residential care facilities has seen little governmental funding and regulation, shifting the responsibility for regulating care labor and care workers largely to the private owners of facilities and employers of the care workers.[14] Formal caregivers' employment arrangements in facilities range from full-time and part-time work, live-in and live-out options in multiple-bed residential care facilities or other assisted residential facilities. With the variance in caregiver arrangements, employment facilities, and the absence of oversight across facilities, the possibilities for exploitation and abuse are expansive.[15] From verbal and emotional abuse, labor exploitation, isolation, retaliation, and wage theft, the lack of labor standard regulation leaves caregivers vulnerable to ill treatment. While the privatized industry of eldercare is booming, the oversight to ensure that workers have basic labor protections in the workplace is weak.[16] As Premilla Nadasen writes, "The care economy parasitically feeds off pain; that is, some people's pain translates into other people's profits."[17]

Research has been done on how to improve the lives and work conditions of Filipino caregivers. Scholars suggest increasing their decision-making power in their daily work routine or providing care workers with ample information about their jobs before they arrive in a new country and when they arrive.[18] Studies show that when agencies and employers specify the job descriptions of care workers and acknowledge that the intrinsic motivation of care workers as a "helping professional," it underplays that this position might also leave workers vulnerable to exploitation in the name of "helping" or "caring" for one's patient.[19] Yet most studies agree that even when localized workplace conditions could be improved, the rate of continued exploitation, without structural change, is impossible. And although this book supports the long-standing evidence regarding workplace violations for caregivers, the focus of this book is laying bare these conditions—and their local and transnational resonances—to provide a basis for continued political organizing, mobilizing, and educating of Filipino migrant care workers.

Why Do So Many Filipinos Work as Caregivers?

For Filipino migrants, securing work as a caregiver has become a stepping-stone to financial stability upon their arrival and transition to the United States. But how did so many of them come to do this work? Filipinos were immigrating to the San Francisco/Bay Area in droves after the Hart-Cellar Act of 1965, which loosened the quota restrictions for many ethnic immigrant groups from Asia and Latin America. In cities like Daly City, which neighbors San Francisco, and the cities in the East and South Bay Area, many Filipino immigrants were answering the call for workers in various professional industries, such as nursing, teaching, and manufacturing, that buttressed the Bay Area's signature booming Silicon Valley technology industries.

But before then, immigrant labor was the foundation of building wealth and whiteness in transforming the rural region into an agricultural industry flanked by racist and oppressive laws.[20] Between the late nineteenth and early twentieth century, businesses in the horticultural industry in large swaths of the Bay Area were managed by white family farms with orchard fruits like apricot and prunes, berries and vegetable crops that relied on Asian labor for harvesting, irrigation, and packing of crops.[21] The marked racial differences between the white owners of Bay Area farms and the Asian immigrant workers, including Filipino seasonal laborers, produced region-specific racialized and class stratification that continues to structure the Bay Area's labor landscape. Yet the transformation of the region's economic focus from agricultural to technological necessarily includes an imposition of state policies that prioritized settler and imperial militarization.

In the 1940s, Silicon Valley's development was at the intersection of military investment, universities, and the federal government.[22] The demand for the production of military technology was key in developing the labor needs in the region.[23] Between 1950 and 1974, hundreds of Silicon Valley firms, funded by the US Department of Defense, cropped up to produce heat-resistant transistors, microchips, semiconductors, and integrated circuitry (for handheld calculators and, later, for electronic weaponry like missile technology, for example). Erstwhile orchards of fruits and vegetables transformed into the establishment of sites for technological research and development with the partnership of public funds, private corporations, and universities, like Stanford University.[24] Studies have shown that the spike in economic development that benefited US military and private corporations imposed great damage to the ecology of the region and to Asian and Latino workers in the blossoming industry.[25] While the innovations in technological development flourished, the then-unknown environmental impacts and effects on workers' health were ignored. Rather, an explosion in technological manufacturing created a need for low-wage work in Silicon Valley. The 1965 Immigration Act, which increased the number of Latino and Asian immigrants, gave way to the required labor that was to power the region's new economic initiatives.

Chain migration ushered in a spike in immigrants from the Philippines, especially to the San Francisco Bay Area. A classic trajectory would be an "anchor migrant," someone who came to work in the States with a visa, earning citizenship and formalizing a petition for parents, siblings, and children who qualified for family reunification. Because the port of San Francisco was so nearby, Daly City became a hub for many Filipino chain migrations into different parts of the Bay Area, including Silicon Valley and its surrounding suburbs, such as Santa Clara, Milpitas, Union City, and Fremont.[26] In this way a pool of available immigrant labor with education, English language capacity, and the need to earn a wage propelled Filipino immigrants to fill gaps in the many industries that required workers. As Filipinos migrated to the Bay Area, they branched out from their anchor ethnic enclave and filled jobs in the manufacturing factories in technology.

In an interview, Jess, a sixty-nine-year-old immigrant working as a caregiver, who came to the United States as a young person in the late 1970s, explained:

> In our community, there are a lot of people who used to work in electronics, who used to work at the big companies. When there was a recession, they had nowhere else to go but become a caregiver. They went into care homes, others did one-on-one, others to day programs. All of those you're considered a caregiver. Yup. And even if they're not considered caregivers, usually there are people in their families who are caregivers, especially in the Filipino community.

In the 1970s and '80s, as the tech industry became emplaced and entrenched in the American national political economy, high-tech workers from Asia immigrated to fill middle-class professions. Yet the need for low-wage labor in manufacturing and assembly persisted. My own family members who immigrated to the Bay Area in the early '80s worked for companies like Sun Microsystems and Texas Instruments in assembly. As neoliberal shifts in American deindustrialization, many manufacturing jobs went to the Global South for cheaper labor and larger profits for technology corporations; therefore, many Filipino migrants in the Bay Area were left to find industries that needed workers.[27]

The increase in the privatization of eldercare after 1965 converged with the opening up of the immigration quotas for countries like the Philippines that ushered in concentrated destination regions like the San Francisco Bay Area and Southern California.[28] Traditional port cities for Filipino immigrants—namely, San Francisco and Los Angeles—boasted some of the highest traffic of Filipino immigrants post-1965. Invoking a multilevel analysis here, it is key to state that the migration of Filipinos to the Bay Area required multiple streams of professional, aspirational, semiprofessional, and low-wage labor. Although some Filipinos came with visas to work as nurses and teachers, the nature of chain migration is that not all migrants would have the same opportunities to ascend into economic mobility and stability. In fact, it was quite the opposite. Migrating to the Bay Area through family petitions required all members of a family to take advantage of labor markets in demand of workers. And in these destination cities of the Bay Area, and through the networks to which they migrated, Filipino migrants found work in industries with high demand and low requirements for qualifications. For newly arrived Filipinos, work opportunities in caregiving traveled through word of mouth in social immigrant networks; with minimal credentials required, Filipino migrants have used caregiving to accrue the capital they sought through labor migration.

Many Filipino migrants find work at residential care facilities, which are nonmedical facilities that provide long-term care and assistance with daily living activities for persons sixty years of age or older, those with developmental disabilities, and those who have chronic illnesses. Caregivers work as both live-out and live-in caregivers, the latter requiring them to live and work at the same facility. Formal caregivers' work consists of helping with activities such as bathing, grooming, toileting, laundry, feeding, cooking, ambulation assistance, house cleaning, sanctioned medical care, patient lifting, and basic companionship.[29] In California there are no specific staff-to-patient ratios, only a vague mandate for residential care facility owners to provide "adequate" staffing. Reports have established that the model for residential care facilities for long-term care for the elderly has poor requirements for inspection frequency, which can result in deleterious effects for both caregivers and the consumers of care.[30] Multiple tenets of the Fair Labor Standards Act are frequently violated by a range of care facilities in denying workers' wages, forcing caregivers to work beyond eight hours, even as staff-consumer ratios increase in care facilities. While complaints about care in facilities are often lost in a broken complaint system, caregivers resort to quitting their jobs or advocating for themselves with the threat of retaliation and termination.[31] Although all care workers are covered under minimum wage and overtime pay protections, caregivers can easily work more than twelve hours a day without proper meal and rest breaks and interrupted sleep in care facilities, which are often private settings.[32]

While some Filipinos, specifically Filipina immigrants, have taken long-term care as an entrepreneurial opportunity, scholars argue that owning and operating residential care facilities can be a contradicting and conflicting experience for Filipinas.[33] Indeed, Filipina care facility owners have extracted profit from care workers, especially fellow Filipinos, however, these dynamics occur under specific neoliberal divestment from state-funded services in long-term care, housing, and community health for the very facilities that are essential to eldercare. While Filipino facility owners and employers are seemingly at odds with their Filipino employees working as caregivers in their facilities, my perspective is that the social class distinction between care home owners and caregivers is mitigated by political and economic systems and processes that devalue the labor in the whole enterprise of caregiving. More importantly, the co-ethnic tensions that arise when Filipino caregivers are mistreated by Filipino employers under any given condition in the labor of care services cannot be *solely* explained by "crab mentality" based on Filipino ethnic and cultural imposition. Rather, I understand these problems of exploitation through the economic necessity that racial capitalism engenders in the United States, specifically on the devaluation of care work. While the political interest of the neoliberal state is to allow the privatization of long-term care, thus allowing Filipino entrepreneurs to corner the market on administrating care homes, Filipinos see their economic opportunity to own care homes as an aspirational class politics to achieve a status that is proximal to whiteness. Still, I will not deny that much of the exploitation that happens among Filipinos relies on negative cultural tenets of obligation and gendered patriarchal logics. However, in this book I hope to tease out the gendered and ethnic tensions among Filipinos and Filipinas in various positions of the caregiver industry. And, more important, I hope to provide the larger context of racial capitalism and the devaluation of domestic labor in the United States to identify how and where Filipino caregivers land in the American racial order.

Many Filipino caregivers endure difficult work conditions in care facilities in order to support their families in the United States and in the Philippines.[34] Their social indebtedness to their employers or to the immigrants who helped them get their jobs, coupled with high financial debt to recruitment agencies or lenders that facilitated their migration, place caregivers in precarious positions. The US caregiving industry's lax regulatory measures produce tremendous instability for them while they are in the country, but before they immigrate it is important to underscore that the political and economic conditions in the Philippines that induce their migration play an important role in why many of them persist in their occupation, no matter the exploitation.

Filipina American scholars Robyn Rodriguez and Anna Romina Guevarra have long established that the Philippines is a "labor brokerage state" that is committed to a historic and continuing system of exporting its citizens and migrant workers to the world.[35] A large percentage of Filipino migrants working abroad take up jobs in the domestic care industry as nannies, housekeepers, caregivers to the elderly, companions, and similar occupations. Cultural traits such as "warm," "caring," and "respectful" to the elderly have been assigned to Filipinos—such rhetoric aims to facilitate the gendered export of care workers.[36] This logic's circulation within the Philippine and its diaspora has had tremendous impact in the preferences of US care recipients for Filipinos. Yet Filipinos' answer to a global demand for care workers also points to the absence of sustainable livelihood in the Philippines, where nurses have been underemployed even in the height of the pandemic.[37] Therefore, understanding why so many Filipinos are caregivers requires a transnational analysis that accepts that their "willingness" or proclivity to caregiving starts even before they leave their home country.[38] A whole history of producing migrant care workers and the continued demand for low-wage care workers can help us build our understanding of why so many Filipinos are caregivers.[39]

Through what Shellee Colen has called "stratified reproduction"—a concept that captures how the ongoing commodification of social reproductive labor amplifies already existing stratification based on race, ethnicity, class, gender, sexuality, especially on a global scale—I intend to start in the place where care workers in the United States, a majority of whom are ethnic immigrant women of color, come from: the Global South. They are conceptualized and targeted as potential low-wage care workers before they even migrate to the United States, Europe, Middle East, and Asia-Pacific.[40] The systemic nature of neoliberal sending states exporting their citizens is not a new idea, but it has been solidified as a characteristic of contemporary globalization.[41] Labor export is vital to the political and economic strategies of developing states to participate in global capitalism.

And in receiving countries like the United States, inequality is central in the American racial order—enshrined by capitalism, as Ruthie Wilson Gilmore has put it—care workers inherit long-standing racialized and gendered histories of devaluation.[42] From Indigenous women and enslaved Africans serving settler colonialists, to imported Chinese "boys" and Asian women trafficked for forced sex work in the early twentieth century, to the racial politics of US imperialism in the Asia-Pacific and West Indies, empire and settler colonization was not only a violent conquest but also a reorganization of domestic life reliant on the servitude of women of color and immigrants.[43] Scholars insist that the key to understanding this historical trend is accepting that the "care labor regime meet up with the racialization of immigrant workers in the labor market generating such precariousness that choice is limited de facto."[44]

Furthermore, in the Filipino community in the Bay Area today, our inherited work in low-wage care industries pulls apart these many scales in tension. The global and transnational scale is enmeshed in the national and historical legacies of how care has always been assumed as cheap, dirty, and the work of "disposable" people in the United States. In my work I've tried to think about linking these various grades of care work through the lens of "social reproductive labor." I introduce this concept in the following section to integrate a Marxist class analysis in the racialization, gendered, and sexualized contexts of global traffic in care.

Why Isn't Caregiving a Sustainable Job?

It is a given that care is a necessary and inevitable part of individual and collective life, yet it has been historically devalued.[45] On a systemic level, contradicting public policies have turned toward home care for elders and people with disabilities, yet political support and funding has not followed suit. While the Americans with Disabilities Act of 1990 and the *Olmstead* decision in 1999 have affirmed that long-term care services should provide the option for home care, long-term services and supports have continued to rely on flimsy and shifting Medicaid and Medicare budgets. Across medical institutions, state legislators, insurance companies, hospitals and medical staff, care home owners and administrators characterized long-term services and support care workers as unskilled and replaceable.[46] One piece of evidence that demonstrates this contemptuous culture against caregivers is the deplorable low wages they receive. It follows that if structural and cultural views of caregivers do not recognize the central role they play in long-term care and in the quality of life of the millions of people they care for, then the workers will bear the brunt of this quandary.

I interpret the devaluation of care work, from eldercare to child care and domestic labor, as a reflection of the contemporary neoliberal, capitalist society we live in. Social reproductive theory provides a theoretical framework to situate the paradoxical experiences of caregivers as essential yet disposable.[47] Early Marxist feminist scholars have examined social reproductive labor to highlight the significant labor processes and practices that produce the worker who in turn surrenders their labor power to contribute to the surplus value of the commodities that keep the public economy thriving.[48] In a particular phase, feminists argued for wages for work done in the home, mostly by women, that was essential in producing the "breadwinners" in the family. By labeling the unpaid work of domesticity as social reproductive labor, scholars asserted that ascribed "women's" work was, in fact, the foundation for the profits accumulated by corporations.[49] In short, it was hard work and housework that exploited women. An important facet of these ideas was that pink-collar sectors in helping professions, retail, teaching, and service were an extension of social reproduction and that such work echoed a similar devaluation, exploitation, and lack of deserved compensation.

A renewed interest in social reproductive theories has been expanding the scope of social reproductive labor as not only sites of exploitation but also possible junctures for political mobilization, thus including the experiences and activisms of women and people of color that encompass fights for housing, education, and health care; political organizing to recognize the work and rights of domestic workers; advocacy for social supports for early childhood care, education, and eldercare; and the efforts to unionize nurses and care staff at hospitals, nonhospital medical institutions, and care facilities for the elderly.[50] An ongoing debate regarding the value-generating potential of social reproductive labor ensues among Marxist feminist scholars; however, in this book it is important to note that I view caregivers' paid employment and the litany of their unpaid care work—for their own families across an ocean and the people they are paid to care for—as labor that generates value, allowing for the accumulation of profit.

Social reproductive labor theories offer us a way to examine not just the labor process that is extracted and devalued under capitalism for caregivers; it also elaborates on the *relationship* between what is valued by the wage and what is essential to the market economy that is at odds with the care and reproduction of life. Moreover, recent social reproductive theory scholars have forged ahead with the insistence that the coproduction of gendered, sexualized, and racialized hierarchies is, in fact, embedded with the bifurcation of value between productive labor and (waged and unwaged) social reproductive labor. Taking this notion to a global and transnational scale, I draw on Shellee Colen's concept of "stratified reproduction" that defines social reproductive labor:

> Physical and social reproductive tasks are accomplished differentially according to inequalities that are based on hierarchies of class, race, ethnicity, gender, place in a global economy, and migration status and that are structured by social, economic, and political forces. The reproductive labor—physical, mental, and emotional—of bearing, raising, and socializing children and of creating and maintaining households and people (from infancy to old age) is differentially experienced, valued, and rewarded according to inequalities of access to material and social resources [and] historical and cultural contexts. Stratified reproduction, particularly with the increasing commodification of reproductive labor, itself reproduces stratification by reflecting, reinforcing, and intensifying the inequalities on which it is based.[51]

In this way, I lean on social reproductive theories to highlight the illogical nature of care as essential and devalued and that this ideology is not just American-centric; rather, it has global reverberations that are constitutive of neoliberalism.[52]

To close this section, I acknowledge that caregiving is not a sustainable job just because of the reasons above but also because the people who need long-term care and support are not valued in our contemporary capitalist culture and society. If the treatment and exploitation of care workers is evidence of the devaluation of their work, we can extend this argument about the lives and well-being of elders, the ill, and disabled people while the support and care they require for daily living is rejected. As Akemi Nishida argues, under the neoliberal US health-care assemblage, "bodies are capacitated and debilitated alongside the flow of Medicaid funds, industry profits, labor capacities and care needs," thereby reducing both care workers and care recipients, and, in fact, the relationship between the two, to one of exploitable opportunity.[53] And although this book will not represent the experiences of the care recipients for the caregivers included in the study, I recognize that the devaluation of both groups under neoliberalism is derived from racism, ableism, sexism, and classism. These social injustices, then, not only describe the parallel contemporary and historical degradation of respect for life and care work; they also create shared stakes in bettering the work conditions of care workers.

Capitalism relies on the extraction and denigration of health from workers, specifically relying on relaxing regulation of occupational health and hazards to keep workers healthy.[54] The maintenance of poor work conditions that extrapolate workers' labor power, across industries, without acknowledgment of workers' holistic health is a part of the rubric of capitalist exploitation. Scholars have argued that the labor process that extracts health from workers is carried out in and through racial inequalities, and the health of caregivers in an underregulated industry is no different.[55]

COVID-19 and the Failure of Privatized Care

Filipino nurses make up 33 percent of deaths from COVID-19 front lines but are only 3 percent of the American nurse workforce. The numbers of deaths from Filipinos across multiple health-care front lines is difficult to gauge, spanning home health aides, certified nurse assistants, and direct care workers. From their hesitance to report their occupations because of undocumented status or a myriad of other reasons, we can only guess how many Filipinos suffered from the lack of protections and funding for frontline health-care workers in residential care facilities, assisted living facilities, and nursing homes. Still, preliminary studies that have examined the impact of the pandemic on Asian American communities in the United States have shown that when disaggregated, the Filipino community suffered disproportionately from COVID-19 deaths compared to other Asian American groups. Although studies have yet to show the correlation, the uneven impact of the pandemic in the Filipino community might be attributed to the number of Filipinos working in the health field on multiple front lines.

During fieldwork I had the opportunity to attend Zoom workshops and meetings with geriatric medicine doctors, professors of medicine, and public health professionals at COVID centers run by the city of San Francisco who were bracing for and, later, reflecting on supporting caregivers in residential care facilities and assisted residential facilities. My field notes reflect that public health professionals' and doctors' experiences demonstrated that caregivers' contraction of and death from COVID-19 were often attributed to the lack of infrastructure to support care workers working in nonmedical settings. Staff at COVID centers lamented that care workers in long-term care facilities were not considered part of the health-care system and therefore suffered more under the lack of access to protections than did their institutionalized counterparts. The invisibility of caregivers can be explained by two reasons. First, the American model of health care narrowly defines health through acute care—in other words, medical conditions are often defined as conditions that can and must be cured with a hospital stay. Therefore, any other types of necessary medical care—for instance, the care necessary after hospital stays or for those who suffer with chronic illness—often remain an afterthought and, dangerously, are unsupported by state funding and social services. This requirement renders nonmedical care and, more important, nonmedical care workers, necessary but largely invisible to the health-care system. In the context of COVID-19, many of the caregivers caring for the elderly were not deemed part of the essential health-care workforce who needed education, training, and protective personal equipment (PPE). Thus, many Filipino caregivers in the Bay Area were not only vulnerable to contracting the virus, but they were also relatively powerless in negotiating for better safety conditions (e.g., PPE) and health provisions (e.g., paid sick leave) with private employers or agencies.

Second, because of the wanton privatization of eldercare and the numerous forms of employment arrangements between those who need care and caregivers, one standard method of disseminating information and PPE was out of reach. In San Francisco, for example, residential care facilities and assisted residential facilities are overseen by the California Department of Social Services and Community Care Licensing, which had no protocol and training to inform administrators of facilities, much less caregivers, about infectious diseases and pandemic control. These state-level departments regulating long-term care are often mismatched in administrating the kind of training that was being administered by the Department of Public Health almost daily at the height of the pandemic. Additionally, the variation in residential care facilities, assisted residential facilities, nursing homes, and one-on-one care arrangements, and state-authorized payment or private pay made it difficult to ensure information regarding COVID-19 was being distributed—and even harder to track—if the information was indeed ending up with direct care workers.

Moreover, many caregivers are undocumented. The characteristic of working as care workers in private homes and settings offers relative safety from US Immigration and Customs Enforcement surveillance and raids, as they can work in small teams and even on their own. State departments and agencies could hardly regulate facilities that employ undocumented workers because facility administrators worked in such secretive terms with their care workers. The pandemic shut down any lines of communications with facilities employing undocumented workers because so many employers or nursing home owners were fearful of being exposed for their labor practices.

Elsewhere, I, along with collaborator Dr. Katherine Nasol, have written that COVID-19 only exacerbated the crisis in caregiving.[56] Before the pandemic, the caregiving industry was rife with labor standard violations, from understaffing, wage theft, lack of proper breaks in the workday, retaliation from employers, and interrupted sleep, to name a few. The pandemic ushered in a dual crisis for caregivers—the toxic ratio of exploitable workers and a global pandemic panic trapped caregivers in their jobs with no way to negotiate for better work conditions. Caregivers from their various work arrangements had little to no collective organization to rely upon for workplace advocacy. The information regarding new pandemic updates were obfuscated by numerous bureaucratic breakdowns. All of these factors resulted in a vulnerable population of essential workers, exposed to the COVID-19 virus with neither workplace protections nor secure benefits for health care. On the question of "Why are caregivers at risk, especially under COVID-19?" the most direct and complex answer is that the systems that are supposed to protect both caregivers and consumers of care services have failed.[57] And, in fact, what Nasol calls the neoliberal governance of care has worked.[58]

And yet, faced with a global pandemic, Filipino caregivers did not back down from their work in caring for the most vulnerable population — and caring for one another. In unearthing the complex web of systematic failures, I also discovered the underbelly of a caregiver mesh network that helped caregivers to retrieve critical information about the COVID-19 virus, provide necessary PPE for lockdown periods, and ensure vital social supports for caregivers at this time. Although I do not propose that this network can supplant any systemic funding and reorganization needed to resolve the open wounds of the caregiving industry, I argue that, for Filipino migrants, the ethics of caregiving extend from their relationship with their consumers. Hence, the kind of radical care they implement is shaped by their caregiving work, a deep sense of responsibility for one another, and for their families in the Philippines.

METHODS AND METHODOLOGY

The research used for this book draws from three different periods of data collection and analysis. Most important, all the research for this book was conducted in collaboration and with participation of many people and organizations. The first phase of data collection and analysis is based on a participatory action research (PAR) project in collaboration with organizations such as the Filipino Community Center, GABRIELA San Francisco, and MIGRANTE San Francisco; scholars like Dr. Robyn Rodriguez; and students from San Francisco State University and the University of San Francisco. Between 2013 and 2014, in what we called "The CARE Project," Dr. Rodriguez and I trained Filipino caregivers and Filipino American students and activists on being critical of the scientific method of research, redefining qualitative methods and social science research as a part of our community's ongoing methods of making sense of our world, and collecting caregivers' stories through *kuwentuhan*. The method of kuwentuhan, a Philippine cultural practice of storytelling that can facilitate the exchange of essential information among its participants, demystified the process of collecting "formal research" that often scared our Filipino migrant participants and collaborators.[59] This PAR project relied on the technological prowess and flexible time and work of Filipino American students and activists who assisted with recording and transcribing. The action portions of the project resulted in a cultural production that depicted the lives of Filipino caregivers, a fact sheet on the wage theft many caregivers experienced, and the formalization of an organization, MIGRANTE San Francisco.

Still, given that this data is dated, the thirty caregivers whose experiences were collected in individual interviews and kuwentuhan sessions are used as consultative background for this book. To prepare this manuscript, I revisited and re-coded the transcribed qualitative data from this first round of data collection with Filipino caregivers in the San Francisco Bay Area to pick up on major themes regarding their work conditions of caregiving. I use these themes to draw through lines between the constant and unchanging characteristics of caregiving in the data collected in the past five years.

Beginning in 2017 and ending in 2019, I received funding from the National Institutes of Health to return to data collection on the lives of Filipino caregivers. I trained and collaborated with undergraduate and graduate students at San Francisco State University to craft a mixed-methods study aimed at examining physical and mental health outcomes among Filipino caregivers in the San Francisco Bay Area. Through survey research we collected information about formal Filipino caregivers' work conditions, such as types of daily living assistance tasks, hours of work, wages, access to wages, wage deductions, meal and rest breaks, sick leave, and access to health insurance and vacation days, or lack thereof. We asked Filipino caregivers to self-report their stress levels using a numerical scale in the same survey to capture their perceptions of their physical and mental health status amid their appraisal of the impact caregiving work had on their emotional life.[60] However, because there is a dearth of validated measures on cultural values of formal caregivers, we created and included questions on sociocultural contexts to learn about how stress levels and caregiving work might be attributed to Filipino caregivers' social ties to their families in the Philippines.

During this phase, we also used *kuwentuhan* to collect qualitative data with a semi-structured guide, but the conversation relied mainly on the Filipino cultural value of talk-story wherein participants could pick up and expound on themes they deemed important. In kuwentuhan, researchers and caregivers could explore deeply how Filipino care workers come to understand and act on their health behaviors at their workplace and in their lives more broadly. In kuwentuhan sessions, which lasted anywhere between forty-five minutes to an hour, we explored the influence of Filipino cultural tenets regarding respect for the elderly on caregivers' approach to their work. We considered how immigrant social networks and Filipino cultural values like *utang ng loob* (social reciprocity) impacted caregivers' feelings of obligation to staying with the jobs procured by their acquaintances and friends. More important, kuwentuhan sessions allowed caregivers to reflect on their own health behaviors while caregiving. These sessions often had one or more caregivers and a researcher (either me or a student researcher) contributing to the discussion.

This pilot phase comprises 114 care workers who lived in the San Francisco Bay Area, ages ranging from eighteen to eighty-five, who answered the surveys and interviews. Among the participants, 78.6 percent self-identified as women and 21.4 percent as men. Additionally, 82.6 percent of participants self-identified as Filipina/o and 15.1 percent as Filipina/o Americans, the latter demarcated if the person was born in the United States. The average time caregivers in this study lived in the United States is 16.2 years. We collected a total of 19 kuwentuhans. With this data, my co-researchers, Elaika Celemen and Kristal Osorio, published a paper arguing that a caregiver's sociocultural contexts, including labor conditions in a privatized US eldercare industry and transnational obligations to families in the Philippines, shape how they perceive their health as it is associated with their formal caregiving work.[61]

Between 2020 and 2021, as the world went into a lockdown in response to the global COVID-19 pandemic—and as I, along with so many, juggled remote teaching and work for my partner and myself, as well as remote schooling for my two young children—I could only think about the Filipino relatives and activists I knew who worked as caregivers. I wondered how the global shift in the world affected them, their health, and their work. But given our mandated conditions of isolation and separation to slow community spread, I had no idea about reaching out to check in with the caregivers in my community, much less design a systematic research study to ascertain their current conditions.

With such prescience, the Carlos Bulosan Center for Filipinx American Studies at the University of California, Davis (UC Davis), under the leadership of Dr. Robyn Rodriguez, revised their "Filipinx Count!" survey to reflect the social shifts that the Filipino American community might have been experiencing under the pandemic. At its outset the survey was designed to create a database of mental and physical health outcomes in the Filipino American community; under its COVID-19 version, the researchers responded to the times and included items such as access to basic needs like food, health care, COVID-19 testing, internet access, financial assistance, and other relevant issues. In collaboration with R. J. Taggueg, a doctoral candidate in sociology at UC Davis and then–research director of the Bulosan Center, we created a version of the "Filipinx Count!" survey for home care workers that measured for mental and physical health outcomes but also explored changes in work conditions and employment and the conditions of Filipino home care workers in their communities and with their families.

We used this survey as a tool to spark a conversation with caregivers and embedded the survey in Zoom kuwentuhans. With my team of student researchers, trained in qualitative data collection alongside the "Filipinx Count!" survey, and with members of the Bulosan Center board, fifty-six surveys were completed and thirty-two kuwentuhans were conducted, fifteen of which we collected under COVID-19 lockdown.

It is important to note that the participatory part in this phase of the research project did not engage Filipino migrant care workers; rather, I collaborated with 1.5- and second-generation Filipino American students to train them on qualitative and quantitative methods, specifically kuwentuhan, and data analysis methods, mainly qualitative, through Zoom sessions. The students in my research group, whom I refer to as "research collaborators," recruited family members and friends to take the survey and participate in kuwentuhan via Zoom. They attended monthly meetings where we would read and discuss articles regarding care work, research methods, and Filipino migration. The action portion of this participatory research culminated in presenting at multiple research conferences together. My research collaborators helped to shape the questions, inquiries, analyses, and dissemination of the research data we collected. I acknowledge that PAR methodology often invites participation of those who are "researched" into the research process, and although my study topic did not reflect the daily realities of Filipino American students and young people, I consider this participatory because many of them engaged in the data collection and analysis of Filipino migrants who are their parents', aunts' and uncles', and grandparents' age cohort. Thus, they were able to ask questions and have conversations about their parents' and grandparents' generation without fear of disturbing the family relations that might otherwise constrict them. In the process, they learned about the difficulty of adapting to a new country and what their own families lived through as immigrants. In the concluding chapter, I explore the potential of intergenerational dialogue through PAR among Filipino migrants and Filipino Americans.

BOOK OVERVIEW

In chapter 1, I introduce ethnographic and qualitative data describing the work conditions of Filipino migrants who are caregivers in residential care facilities for the elderly, assisted residential facilities, and in one-on-one care arrangements. In detail, I examine the daily tempo and tasks of Filipino caregivers wherein they assist their consumers in daily living activities, noting that these work conditions document the existing crisis for eldercare workers. I analyze how caregivers intertwine their daily decisions as workers in, at times, exploitative conditions with their families in the Philippines in mind. This chapter's central argument is that the compounding crisis of underregulation of the caregiving industry along with the transnational responsibilities of caregivers to their families in the Philippines produce what I am calling the "caregivers' contradiction," or in their words, the "no work, no pay" situations they find themselves in.

In chapter 2, I explore the invisibility of caregivers as essential frontline workers during the span of the COVID-19 lockdown and reintegration. With qualitative data from kuwentuhan sessions, I explain the stressors that compounded the already existing crisis of labor for caregivers. Through the unprecedented global and national health pandemic, caregivers found themselves working with people who were the most vulnerable to the COVID-19 virus—those over the age of sixty-five with preexisting health conditions. Their workplaces became hot spots for coronavirus transmission, which then put them, their families, and their communities at high risk. Yet, this sector of frontline workers often remained excluded from the popular narrative of the traditional hospital-setting frontline workers and, more important, out of the conversations of workplace safety protections. Moreover, Filipina/o care workers faced blatant racism and discrimination in their interactions with patients that arose from the moral panic that echoed historic "master narratives" labeling their "yellow" bodies as carriers of disease. I argue that this dual crisis in the caregiving industry worked within the neoliberal schema of placing individual responsibility on caregivers to protect themselves and their families and communities.

Building on my past book, *The Labor of Care*, I extend my theory of "communities of care" to explore how caregivers defined individual, interpersonal, and organizational forms of care for themselves in chapter 3. With the absence of structural support, caregivers expanded existing methods of mutual aid before and during the COVID-19 pandemic. With constraints on gathering and mobility, many caregivers felt isolation and anxiety during the pandemic, yet they relied on forms of religiosity, technological communication, and community organizations to receive and provide essential workplace protections such as PPE and social support through difficult conditions.

In chapter 4, I take the opportunity to reflect on methods and the methodology of the research in this book as a process wherein generations in Filipino America can understand themselves and one another. As a 1.5-generation Filipina American, one who came to the United States as a child and has spent a majority of her life here, I straddle a unique perspective of biculturality and belongingness to both the Filipino immigrant experience and a Filipino American sensibility. My work as an activist, scholar, writer, educator, and community member has always been ensconced in the interstices of many generations—both in immigrant waves and in age cohorts. This chapter lays bare the possibilities and limits of conducting social science research in community, a vulnerability to which I have always been committed in my scholarship. I sustain a discussion about a method I have developed in my work called kuwentuhan, a Filipino practice of talk-story, to think through intergenerational dialogue and activism.

In the epilogue, I report on what has happened in the lives of Filipino migrant workers, including caregivers and the next generation of Filipino Americans as the COVID-19 pandemic continues. I reflect on the abundance of care in the lives of Filipino migrants in the eldercare industry: the care work in their daily jobs, the care they give to their families in the Philippines from afar, and the communities of care they tend to in the United States. I pair that with a discussion of the promise of radical care in the contemporary social movements led by migrant women domestic workers in California. Finally, I leave you with questions and provocations to build the future of care we all deserve.

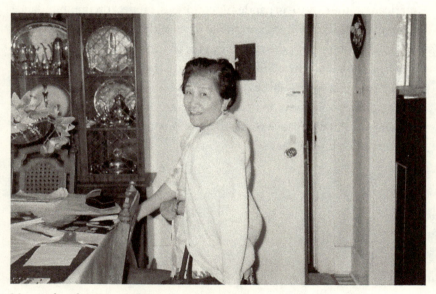
My grandmother Remedios Luna Francisco, ca. 1993

CHAPTER 1

NO WORK, NO PAY

Her clients loved her. Remedios Luna Francisco was their caregiver. And Remedios was my grandmother, my caregiver too, my family, and I called her Nanay—"mother" in Tagalog. She was five feet tall, slender, with soft, wrinkled hands, and brown eyes with cataracts, lightened by her sixty-five years of life, migrations, seven children, and more than twenty grandchildren. She kept her wavy hair short in a pixie cut she would trim herself. Pink rollers would go in every night to keep a tight curl in her hair throughout the workday since the natural curl left years ago. Every morning she would wake up at 5:30 a.m. to start preparing breakfast for the six elderly and developmentally disabled clients in her care home. But before she stepped out onto the kitchen floor to begin her day, she would take out the rollers, draw in her eyebrows, and dab on a little lipstick. As she smacked her lips together, she would turn to me and say, "Always nice to look a little presentable, Val." Even though her workday consisted of staying inside, mostly cooking and cleaning the six-bed care home she worked and lived in, maybe a little gardening in the back or front yard, Remedios made sure she put on her best face, her best self to care for her clients. They loved her for it. I loved her for it.

Right at 6:00 a.m. each day, a parade of elderly and disabled people would start to emerge from their bedrooms on the side of the house that had been turned into a residential care facility. They would commence their morning ritual over the coffeepot, coffee already brewed, with mugs, creamer, and sugar out and ready to be mixed in. Silver-haired clients—all white, most over seventy—would take cups back to the living-room area, where each of them had a spot they had designated as their own. Uncle Harry on one side of the brown plaid couch and Auntie Sheila on the other end, unfolding the crisp morning newspaper. Auntie Elizabeth and Auntie Nancy, clients who lived with Down syndrome and developmental disabilities, respectively, taking their seats on the green couch, sometimes together, sometimes apart. Uncle Jim, an elderly man with developmental disabilities, on an armchair facing the big sliding doors overlooking the backyard. Uncle Joe, a loquacious mover and shaker in his time, perched on his high stool, next to the end of the countertop where Remedios was buttering bread or cutting fruit, chatting away. Two of my siblings and I—all under eleven years old, who lived in the care home—referred to them with the honorifics "uncle" and "auntie," just as we would address elders in the Filipino culture with "*tito*" or "*tita*." They didn't mind at all. We didn't mind either.

At 6:15 a.m. the residents would shuffle over with their coffee cups to the dining table, where I had already set the table with placemats, folded napkins, forks and knives, plates, and glasses for water or juice. Remedios would check to see when all were seated to bring over the hot breakfast on big serving plates. She would float across the kitchen to the dining table singing a melodic, "It's breakfast time!" And then the toast, eggs, and sausages would disappear from the communal plates in a matter of seconds. As her clients ate, Remedios would start another round of Filipino breakfast cooking for me and my two siblings and my grandfather, Porfirio. After her patients wrapped up breakfast, they would head to their rooms to get dressed and prepare for their various day program schedules, family visits, and recreational activities. And it would be time for Remedios's grandkids—me, my little sister, and our older brother—to eat quickly and get on with our day as well.

After breakfast Remedios would clear the table, wash and dry the dishes, and sweep the floors. When the kitchen and dining rooms were tidied, her clients would come back to the counter, which by now had been transformed into a medication distribution center. Remedios had each client's set of medications in separate and neatly hand-labeled baskets. Each of the baskets had a pillbox with each day of the week stamped atop the lids. She would call their names: Harry, Sheila, Elizabeth, Nancy, Joe, Jim. They would have a glass of water or juice to drink down their meds. Then off they went, each having a designated pickup time on some days. On other days, a different collection of them would stay at the facility. She juggled each client's family visit schedules, doctor's appointments, and day programs, along with transport on a weekly basis. When they were away at their daily activities, she would get started with cleaning their rooms. She would turn the beds down, collect their laundry, vacuum, and dust. She would clean the bathrooms, sweeping and mopping the floors and cleaning the toilets and showers until the whole house smelled of Pine-Sol, the unmistakable cleaning agent for floors. Then she would load laundry while a pile of freshly clean clothes from the dryer would get folded. A bit before noon, it would be time to prepare lunch for the clients who were home or on the way home. She would harvest and chop vegetables that she grew in the backyard: spinach, tomatoes, carrots, and zucchini. A vegetable soup on some days, a fresh salad on other days, ham and cheese sandwiches with chips on the weekends. All of these recipes she learned from cookbooks, which she picked up at the Salvation Army, a secondhand store she found near the care home when she first immigrated to Concord, California, in 1986, a trove of "American" culture she could learn about through books and magazines. After all, the kind of vegetable soup she liked, *pinakbet*, was too "exotic" for her American clients' palette, too salty with the fermented shrimp, too strange with the bitter melon and long green beans mixed with kabocha squash that none of them had ever seen before. So it was always spinach, carrot, and zucchini soup—for them.

After lunch, clients would turn to their bedrooms for an afternoon rest. The ones who came home from their day programs would go straight to their rooms for either a nap or a bit of television or reading. Sweet relief. Finally, Remedios had some time to herself. She would mend tattered clothes or work on a dress pattern for me and my little sister. She would go into the backyard and check on the plum trees or the fig tree, gathering some as a treat for us and her clients. Or she might take her prayer book and read to herself for some fleeting moments in the backyard. But not for too long. At 3:00 p.m. clients started to come out of their restful slumber and head back into the living room. Remedios would entertain them by bringing out board games, juggling that with dinner preparation. More chopping or preparing chicken à la king with the leftover wheat slices smashed into muffin tins and toasted in the oven. At 5:00 p.m. she would set the table again: placemats, folded napkins, soup spoons, forks and knives, glasses, and coffee cups. Right at 5:30 p.m. the familiar melody of "It's dinner time!" would coax her patients to the dining table. As she cooked her second dinner, the Filipino food one, her clients would take from the communal plates and remark, "*Ray-me*, this is such a delicious dinner!" They shortened Remedios to "Reme," with an American singsong accent. At 6:30 p.m. Remedios would wheel a television set into the living room, where everyone sat in their seats to watch a bit of *Wheel of Fortune* and *Jeopardy*, and by 8:00 p.m. they would retire to their bedrooms. The end of a day in Reme's care.

But it was far from the end of her workday. Remedios would promptly do the cleaning and prepare meals for the next day. She would ensure all the medications were lined up. She would telephone the care home owner a grocery list and the maintenance requests she had. She would feed us her *menudo*, *pinakbet*, and her *sinigang* with rice. She would help us with our homework and ensure we had our outfits ready for school the next day. At 9:30 p.m.—sometimes later—she would finally fall into her own bed. We three looking up at her from the comforters we had laid out on the floor beside her. She would be asleep in minutes, and as I lulled myself to sleep, I wondered, If Nanay was that tired, what did she dream of?

TRANSNATIONAL OBLIGATIONS AND THE "FILIPINO WORK ETHIC"

My grandmother's daily schedule was packed. To oversee care for six clients and three grandchildren meant she was working and caring nonstop on a regular day. And for many Filipino immigrants working as caregivers, this type of relentless care work—whether it is with their clients or for their family—has been codified as a "Filipino work ethic" by many caregivers in our community. Asked about the intensity of work in her job as a caregiver, Sheila, an immigrant woman in her fifties with adult children and grandchildren in the Philippines, said:

> You have patience if you want to work as a caregiver because you will not like all the jobs. Not all jobs will be easy. And all the jobs you do is one right after the other, nonstop. They should learn about it first before just going straight to work without knowing your rights or the people you can reach out to. Sometimes we aren't given the chance to talk to each other so we aren't aware of how to do the work and we are working too hard. Only have our family in the Philippines in mind. So we work and work, until you are sick or you can't do it anymore.

Sheila attests to the intensity of work as a caregiver, noting that the work can be so taxing that it can lead to negative health issues. Sheila's opening comment regarding patience is a sustaining principle that draws from a Filipino cultural value, *tiis*, or a resolute attitude with a purpose in mind. For Sheila and other migrants, that purpose is to support one's family in the Philippines. Tiis coupled with patience and endurance becomes a narrative for many migrant workers beyond the eldercare industry; however, it is also a contradictory practice for workers providing care to clients while also sacrificing their own health. The patience to "work and work," as Sheila notes, jettisons her work ethic in a transnational context (e.g., for her family), yet she alone has to deal with the health and personal consequences. Mirroring the experience of Remedios's workday, the intertwined strands of "domestic labor," both paid and unpaid, and obligations to biological kin in the Philippines becomes a crucial factor in understanding the lives of Filipina/o caregivers.

In fact, a popular narrative circulated about Filipino caregivers is that their dutiful work ethic and commitment to their patients is the key feature that demonstrates that they are elite care workers.[1] "Work ethic" implies a standard of work behavior adopted by a worker to excel at their occupation, thus providing the worker entitlement to their wage. In the United States, this work ethic is reified as a natural racial, ethnic, or cultural trait for immigrants and people of color in low-wage industries, such as domestic work, agriculture, and other types of urban manual labor like construction. Yet this problematic narrative does not take into account specific sociocultural contexts that drive the work conditions of low-wage workers, especially Filipina/o care workers. In this chapter, I explore the entangled responsibilities of domestic work for these care workers that often produce an exhausting tempo of labor that relies on both a hyperlocal charge of their occupation and a transnational obligation to their families in their proximity and in the Philippines. In what follows, I bridge multiple disciplinary fields on care work to provide a basis to think through the sociocultural contexts for Filipina/o care workers. Then, with quantitative and qualitative data, I demonstrate that the transnational connections of these caregivers are quite present for them in their daily decisions in their care work. I end the chapter offering readers a sense of the schedules, tempo, and intensity of labor in the days of caregivers.

As African American studies scholars in public health and gerontology, Sharon Wallace Williams and Peggye Dilworth-Anderson have studied the dynamics among African American family members who care for their relatives without pay, otherwise called "informal caregivers."[2] They argue that the field responsible for examining caregiving often pays less attention to the racial, cultural, and societal conditions under which African Americans are providing care to their family members, thus undertheorizing why this group of care providers experience such negative health outcomes as caregivers. They propose that frameworks of the "sociocultural, situational, interpersonal, temporal and personal contexts in which they give care" must be made clear before scholars can analyze the work ethics of African American caregivers and, more important, the health consequences of their care work. In fact, they argue that (1) racial ethnic contexts have direct influences on how caregivers provide care, and (2) if interventions are proposed to ameliorate the negative emotional effects of caregiving, these changes must incorporate caregivers' specific sociocultural contexts — in other words, the cultural beliefs and attitudes of caregivers when it comes to providing care to their families. I build on this rich work of African American scholars at the intersection of public health, gerontology, and sociology and apply this theoretical framing to formal Filipino caregivers, those who are providing paid care for elderly and chronically ill clients. I find this theoretical framework useful as Filipino caregivers inherit a racialized and gendered history of domestic work in this country, eldercare notwithstanding.[3] Further, I extend this frame to encompass the transnational imaginary and material obligations Filipino migrants live and work under as formal caregivers. In many ways, their paid labor as workers is enmeshed with their unpaid, transnational responsibilities to their families in the Philippines—two of the chief reasons why many Filipinos migrate to work abroad. Seemingly an individual rationale, scholars have noted that Philippine labor migration is codified through global racial ideologies of domestic labor.[4]

In fact, feminists scholars of color and theorists writing on "social reproductive labor" have argued that hierarchies in gender, race, and ethnicity were specifically organized to privilege whiteness and relegate women of color, poor women, and immigrant women into devalued positions of low-wage domestic work.[5] The entrenchment of a gendered division of domestic labor—separating societal responsibilities between a masculinized public sphere and a feminized private sphere—perpetuated women's work in the home as subordinate. And as white middle-class women surged into the workforce in the mid-twentieth century, the void in domestic work was filled by paying women of color, immigrants, and poor women to fulfill gendered responsibilities.[6] It is important to note that I unfetter care work from the realm of the private sphere into a more general idea of paid care work that includes what Johanna Brenner and Barbara Laslett consider social reproductive labor consisting of "various kinds of work—mental, manual and emotional—aimed at providing the historically and socially, as well as biologically, defined care necessary to maintain existing life."[7] The gendered and racialized nature of domestic work, both waged and unwaged, has undoubtedly shaped US labor demands and the demographic shift for these care workers.[8]

Together, these theoretical frames inform how I will analyze the "work ethic" that has become the linchpin for Filipinos as the "best" kinds of caregivers as an inherited legacy of racial capitalism and gendered social reproductive labor in the United States. My aim for this chapter is to demonstrate a day in the life of Filipino caregivers and to explore what they consider a strong work ethic. I argue that what is normalized as a Filipino caregiver's work ethic can become the normalization of exploitation in caregiving. I pair the dynamics of transnational pressures on migrant workers and the rapacious gendered nature of caregiving work in discussing why Filipinos continually work beyond their health capacities. These coupled social factors and work conditions uphold the problematic narrative of them as the "best" kind of caregivers. I question the idea of "best" care worker because I find that the circulation and internalization of this narrative puts workers at risk while the recognition of their work, in terms of rights and compensation, does not match the labels hoisted on them. The sociocultural contexts and gendered analysis are key in understanding how Filipino caregivers submit to exploitation in their workplaces, and how, structurally, their welfare is betrayed by the lax nonenforcement of labor standards in the caregiving industry.[9]

Home Is Where the Remittances Go

In a survey conducted with Filipino caregivers between 2017 and 2019, my study found that 60 percent of participants reported that their families in the Philippines rely on their income for basic living needs. In a list of reasons about their motivations for migration, 88 percent of caregivers in the same study stated that they migrated to improve their families' lives in the Philippines while searching for better opportunities in the United States. Additionally, 86 percent reported that their migration to the States was based on finding employment. These findings support the extant literature in Filipino American and Filipino diasporic studies where scholars provided the evidence regarding the economic reasoning for Filipino labor migration.[10] And although decisions to migrate extend far beyond economic necessity, it is worth noting that economics remains a driving force and a constraining influence in the lives of Filipino migrants.

Given that many Filipina/o care workers consider their financial responsibility to their families in the Philippines as an intrinsic motivator to work, many care workers disregard their own health and wellness to continue working. A repetitive phrase that rang across interviews and *kuwentuhan*—or talk-story—sessions with multiple Filipina/o migrants was "No work, no pay!" This logic accepts that every day of paid labor means one has something to send home, in terms of remittances, to their family members in the Philippines. Therefore, when asked about her family in the Philippines and how it relates to her work as a caregiver in the United States, fifty-five-year-old Hester, who supports two children in the Philippines, replied, "There's a saying, 'You can't get sick,' *diba*? Not that you won't, but you can't, right? That's a sacrifice you promised to yourself and your family." I point to Hester's reference to her transnational conditions, which are inseparable from how she approaches her work ethic as a caregiver. Essentially, this is the caregiver's contradiction—a promise to family members in the Philippines that contributes to the aforementioned Filipino work ethic wherein many caregivers face the strenuous nature of their occupation and are unable to refuse work because of their obligations. Many caregivers weigh their decision to go to work, above all, against the responsibilities they have to their kin in the Philippines.

Che, a migrant in her late fifties who left one adult child, her spouse, and her aging parents in the Philippines, discussed how the tenet of "no work, no pay" shapes her approach to caregiving:

> *Oh, siempre nag iingat rin kami lalo na sa lifting, kailangan mag ingat.* Of course, we all take good care, especially when lifting. What do "they" say, *bawal magkasakit*, we cannot get sick! (laughs) *So pag kayo nagkasakit, pag hindi nagingat, nay, papano kayo?* We must take good care. Because we don't have the health insurance. Because if we get sick, if we don't take care, *ikaw ang magbabayad pagnagkasakit kayo*, it's you that will pay if you get sick or hurt. *Meron sabihin*, there's a saying: no work, no pay.

The onus is on the worker to maintain their health and safety. Che reminds us of the type of mental preparation and wherewithal migrant workers need to have in order to approach their daily work. Many times in this excerpt, Che refers to a generalized "other" that has taught her how to conceptualize her own health at her workplace—noting what "they" say or remembering a saying about work conditions, she is echoing an idea of how to survive as a caregiver. And in no uncertain terms, she equates this ethic of immaculate and unfailing health to her ability to earn a wage. "No work, no pay" means that Filipino care workers must think of preventing aches, pains, strains, and illnesses as an active exercise in their daily routines—not only because time off will cost a worker their wage but also because they do not have access to health insurance through their employment. Although

Che's reference to a lack of health insurance was a secondary thought in this excerpt, it is important to note that the conditions of many caregivers, as is true for a majority of domestic workers in the United States, are that they do not have basic labor rights such as paid leave, sick time, and access to health insurance.[11] For caregivers, their everyday workplace is a minefield, where they themselves manage and maintain safe working conditions in order to continue to be able to earn a wage without access to proper health care if they do get hurt or sick. Still, what governs many workers' desire to maintain a healthy laboring body is their need to send money to the Philippines.

Whether they have cold symptoms or aches and pains, the decisions Filipina/o caregivers make about going into work is tethered to their responsibilities to their families in the Philippines. When asked if she had incurred any injuries at her job, Richelle, a caregiver for ten years, said:

> It's back pain! Here [gesturing at her lower back]. I injured my back from lifting. And just recently I was doing that. We have a rehabilitation for my knee, because the PT [physical therapist] said I twisted my knee, and I didn't know it. So, I mean, you get hurt, you can't help it. It's the nature of the job. But whenever we assist, even if you do bodily economics, you're really bound to hurt yourself. It's the wear and tear. You know, if you keep on doing something, like, over and over again, you're bound to, you know, injure, have an injury, one or two injuries minor. Yeah.
> Sad, but yeah, nothing you can ever prevent that.

Richelle describes the pain of working with patients where she makes repeated motions, such as lifting or turning. She acknowledges that the nature of her job is that her body goes through "wear and tear" and that, in fact, even if one is aware of how they are moving their bodies during lifting or repetitive motions, there is still no way to prevent injury. Yet, when I asked her about maybe taking time off, especially with physical therapy, to nurse her injuries back to health, Richelle scoffed. "I wish! If I don't work, I don't have a check! You just do what you can to prevent the injury. You just do what you can with the pain. Then you go to work!" Richelle said that her experience with workplace injuries cannot take precedence over the wage she earns as a caregiver.

Few people shared their strategies to keep illnesses and strains away considering a "no work, no pay" ethos. Michelle, a caregiver at a residential care facility who assists in lifting clients in and out of their seated positions to standing and lying down, mentioned that it was important to her to ensure that she could attend to her clients' needs safely. "I have my two daughters in college back in Manila. So when I'm working, all I'm thinking of is how I can do my work to help my patients, but I also don't want to get hurt lifting the heavier ones. My daughters rely on me, that's why." Michelle's concern about the physical aspect of her job is multidimensional: a need to attend to her clients' needs and to be as safe as possible doing her work, with her daughters' stability as the background context informing these decisions. As we engaged in kuwentuhan about how she could prevent injuries, she said:

> For the work, we have to have a certificate for first aid, at least the basics. And then every year we have to watch all these videos; it says it's a requirement of the licensing, all these videos. A lot of them. But after those really basic things, I go to YouTube with my coworkers on the downtime. YouTube clips where they show how to lift, how to do this, and how to do that. We watch together because some of us have never done this kind of work before. Like me, I'm a social worker in the Philippines. When my coworkers told me about the videos, I feel like I'm learning how to work my body and not get hurt.

Michelle's discussion about the resource sharing in her workplace via instructional videos demonstrates one way that caregivers are filling in for absent workplace safety training. Outside of basic first aid and CPR skills, the fact that caregivers are trading strategies to avoid getting hurt demonstrates that many of them share a concern about staying safe doing their jobs. A part of this exchange also demonstrates the acceptance of the risks of getting injured or hurt, thus requiring many of these caregivers to be creative in leveraging the resources they have on the internet to mitigate those risks.

The concept of "no work, no pay" becomes a guiding philosophy around maintaining health and safety; it is also a point of worker solidarity. In a kuwentuhan session with five Filipina caregivers ranging from their late forties to early sixties who were members of the Pilipino Association of

Workers and Immigrants (PAWIS), there was a robust discussion about teaching one another correct techniques for lifting and shifting clients with the purpose of staying uninjured:

ALMA: For example, when you have to turn down if they're bed bound. So you have to turn them every two hours [when you] are changing the diapers. You have to roll them side to side. So that requires, really—push and lift, so, so it depends, on how much you know how to do that.

PINKY: But as caregivers, we should learn the right techniques. You know, to really do it properly. So you'll, you'll not experience pain. So there's always the technique and doing it, but how do you find that out? The techniques that can avoid, you know, you will strain on your shoulder, your arms, your back.

ALMA: Of course, and you know you'll be standing with another caregiver. *Tayo tayo lang, magabiso sa isa't isa.* [It depends on us to give each other the advice on how to do it.] You have to work together to do the heavy lifting, the repeating standing and sitting, so it's easier for all.

RAE: So that's my, my experience and I know some of my friends. *Si Tita Alma at Tita Pinky ang nagturo sakin, kung paano talaga magbuhat para di masaktan kasi nga pagna-injure, no work, diba?*] [It's Tita Alma and Tita Pinky who taught me how to lift so that you don't get her because, right, if you get injured, no work, right?] Then, *no pay.*

The daily exchange in tactics to increase work efficacy within coworkers is one strategy deployed to protect one another's laboring bodies. For the intent of attending to their clients, caregivers acknowledge that they must be one another's on-the-job trainers and teachers. While they might not be certified in body mechanics and lifting clients, they must rely on one another to be able to care for their clients. Still, Rae's comment in this excerpt points to the fact that these safety precautions are not just a concern about physical injury but are also undergirded with preventing a loss in wage if a strain or injury occurs on the job. Without access to health insurance and workers' compensation, caregivers ramp up their on-the-job training and attention to safety as they care for their clients. These same caregivers share the regular routine of remitting funds to their families in the Philippines; therefore, building strategies to stay safe can be understood as a commitment to transnational obligations.

From the same aforementioned survey, I found that 70 percent of caregivers answered that their migration was tied to improving the future of the children in the family, and 73 percent sought to improve the life of their families and look for better opportunities. This sociocultural context of transnational families is a governing principle in how Filipina/o caregivers create their work ethic and approach to the sometimes-difficult working conditions they face. I posit that these transnational contexts are imperative in producing the conditions wherein Filipino caregivers decide to work nonstop, to take up a part-time caregiving job on their days off, or to work a double shift in one day. In my mixed-method study before the COVID-19 pandemic, 81.7 percent of caregivers replied that they had one or more caregiving jobs at any moment. Linda said, "I have many jobs. I work twelve hours for three days, and I can have like two one-on-one patients—traveling on my four-hour break in between, for over six days. I do that because I help my sisters. I have nieces who are going to college for nursing." Like many others, Linda maximizes her time by figuring out how to stack her days with an opportunity to earn as much as she can. The logic by which she does this is guided by her transnational responsibility to fund her nieces' education, save for various projects she has in mind for her home in a Philippine province, and pay her bills here in the United States. The concept of time as a series of opportunities to make money means that Filipino migrants' health must either be looked after vigilantly or ignored all together.

Leif, a one-on-one caregiver whose work schedule varies week to week given his clients' needs, works at a gas station and a fast-food restaurant on evenings and the weekends. He stated, "Kailangan maximize ang oras dito kas nga mga anak sa Pilipinas, may anak at magulang sa Pilipinas. Maraming gastos. Kaya dapat marami din trabaho [I need to maximize my time here because I have children in the Philippines; I have parents in the Philippines. Lots of bills. That's why you have to work a lot too]." Migrants' ability to find opportunities to earn a wage so that they can send money back to the Philippines means they must maintain an ability to show up for one or more jobs daily. For Leif, the costs of being the only person in the United States for his immediate family and family of origin motivates him to work as a caregiver and seek part-time opportunities on his days off. The types of decisions about where to work, what type of work to do, and how much to work is governed by their responsibilities to their families back home. Leif continues, "Ang kailangan lang, dedication. Isa, papano na treat mo ang matanda nasa iyo, respeto. Tapos, dedication sa pamilya. Tuloy tuloy ang trabaho, wag alalahin ang sarili, kasi nga, no work, no pay [What you need is dedication. One, how you treat your elderly clients that you're in charge of, respect. Then, dedication to your family. Gotta work and work, just don't worry about you, because if not, no work, no pay]."

Leif's multiple jobs during his time off as a caregiver is informed by what he sees as continued "dedication" to a larger purpose of supporting his family. However, spliced in the middle of his comments is a short dismissal of himself and his health, "don't worry about you," or in Filipino, *wag alalahin ang sarili*, can be interpreted as selflessness and altruism. However, in the context of kuwentuhan, Leif's train of thought stemmed from earning a wage and maximizing his time for his family, which meant he didn't have time or the need to worry about his own wellness. In this way, Leif's concern about his clients and his family, everyone but himself, is a way to keep his purpose sharp and at the forefront of his mind—which also means he will ignore his own health if it means being able to go into work that day.

In fact, in the mixed-method study on the health outcomes of Filipina/o caregivers conducted within the COVID-19 pandemic, my research shows that almost all caregivers would underreport negative health outcomes. We found this in our surveys, where 31 percent of participants reported that they did not experience pain or injury from their jobs. However, in the subsequent interviews reflecting on the surveys, most of the participants would pause after this question and say a version of "Well . . . there was this one time" or "No pain at all . . . except for." For example:

VALERIE: Is there persistent pain in your body—for example your hands, shoulders, knees?
SERENA: No, not at all.
VALERIE: Okay.

SERENA: (Few seconds of silence) Well... actually. We get hurt every time, you really can't stay away from it. Especially when you have a client who's really, umm, active. When he grabs you, there's a scratch. It's included in the job. It's included in the job.

Another instance:

VALERIE: How about persistent pain in your body—for example, hands, shoulders—
CHARYLLE: Mm, no. Not really.
VALERIE: Not really, okay.
CHARYLLE: (Silence) Nothing like that, but sometimes I have joint pain. Especially when you're standing and assisting all day. It's painful.

A last example:

VALERIE: Is there persistent pain in your body?
PURI: Oh, no. Not at all. But only just my shoulders. And there's tension in my back. But only when I work too much.

I include this trio of exchanges to demonstrate the hesitation Filipina caregivers display when talking about their health and wellness. In the first example, Serena's comment about the pain being "included in the job" is the operative phrase in these exchanges. Caregivers are interpreting their pain and health outcomes as part of their work, not worthy of note. Especially not worthy of time off from their jobs. Quickly after these exchanges, I would acknowledge the pain caregivers had incurred, investigate if the pain came from the motions or actions in their jobs, and then I would ask if they felt like they could go to a doctor and take time to remedy their injuries. "Well, no work, no pay, you know," said Charylle. It was a pointed end to my line of inquiry.

Caregivers' health and wellness, or the deterioration of such, seemingly weighs less than the responsibilities many caregivers have to their families in the Philippines. While scholars have shown that workers' self-reported health outcomes underestimate the types of health conditions they experience, my mixed-method study produced diverse results.[12] The qualitative data displayed that many caregivers, albeit reticent, experienced various negative outcomes, yet the quantitative surveys found that they scored under or nearly the same in comparison to other "care workers" in the United States. Curious about these findings, I interpret this pivot in the kuwentuhan or interview sessions as linked to the logic of "no work, no pay."

Interpreting Filipino Caregivers' Self-Reported Health Outcomes

In our kuwentuhan, even with caregivers explicitly discussing work conditions that put their health at risk, the survey results produced contradicting findings about caregivers' self-reported health outcomes. When asked about the status of their emotional health as a caregiver, survey analyses indicate that caregivers appear to be emotionally healthy on measures of purposefulness and feeling worthy and valuable in their work. In total, 96 percent of participants responded positively to the question asking if they "experienced deep fulfillment in their life" as care workers.

My research team was confounded with the findings regarding mental health outcomes given that the survey contradicted care workers' self-reported physical health outcomes. This paradox further belied the basic working conditions such as regular breaks across the workday, meal breaks, and uninterrupted sleep, which we found were frequently violated. Additionally, 64 percent of participants reported that their breaks were cut short, and 25 percent reported that both clients and employers have interrupted even their off-hours time. Furthermore, 58 percent of live-in care workers did not have a sleeping space of their own, often sharing with clients and other staff, and 33 percent reported they did not sleep in a proper bed, with care workers reporting the multiple ways that their workplace set up hazardous environments.

The results for self-reported physical health outcomes told a different story. Sixty percent of caregivers in our study self-reported various symptoms of physical exhaustion, and 39.4 percent self-reported that they had "difficulty making decisions" in the measures we used for stress indicators. These two factors often point to depression and anxiety. Our data showed that 68.7 percent of caregivers reported feeling ill at some point during their work hours, and 52.4 percent reported feeling exhaustion after their workday. Hence, in descriptive analysis, the contradiction between mental and physical health outcomes did not allow us to support a correlation between negative physical health outcomes based on the working conditions of Filipino care workers.

Still, I propose that lack of significance and inconsistency in the data could be attributed to perceptions of stress impacted by sociocultural factors and transnational contexts. Drawing from a "culture-centered approach" as an analytical frame specifically with health outcomes and migrant workers, I argue that these mixed findings are partly a result of migrant care workers underrepresenting their stress and health ailments because (1) they are precarious workers in an unforgiving industry, and (2) they are migrants with transnational family dependents.[13] Next I discuss these two aspects as they contribute to the findings concerning health outcomes in my research. These sociocultural contexts are key in understanding how the health of Filipino care workers is affected, thus explaining the contradiction in the quantitative and qualitative data in the study.

NORMALIZED EXPLOITATION AND COVID-19

I have hesitated to call caregiving an "industry" in the past because I wanted to valorize the work of care beyond the scope of capital, and I feared that calling this profession an industry would reduce the layers and textures of care work by caregivers into mere economic units. But as much as I resisted, the word and mechanics of an industry based on profit and exploitation kept bringing me back to this word and, more important, this dynamic. In this section, I demonstrate the precarity produced by the mechanisms in which eldercare should be considered an industry—that is, I join it to a Marxian analysis that marks the work of caregiving with flexibility and disposability.[14] Coupled with US abandonment of the welfare state, caregivers cannot insist on caring for themselves when they fall ill or when they experience workplace injuries. "No work, no pay" is no longer just a demonstration of the Filipino work ethic; rather, it is produced through the constraints of a caregiving industry that is driven by profit and not guided by concern for quality care for clients nor worker welfare.

Beyond the economic metrics of industry profits, I argue that the caregiving industry's schemes of flexibility and disposability are undergirded by race and ethnicity, gender, and status of immigration, where these nodes become the levers in which work inequalities are pulled and pushed. Moreover, the political trends of neoliberal divestment in social welfare, specifically away from long-term care for the elderly and ill, produce the conditions for varying private and semiprivate enterprises that are difficult to regulate and standardize to protect workers' rights.[15] Caregiving has a high demand for care workers, yet it is an invisible industry given that the work of caregiving has a multitude of permutations in terms of obtaining work, maintaining and securing stable employment, and the types of full- and part-time care arrangements. Filipino caregivers have said they secure work as caregivers in three ways: through informal immigrant networks, with employment agencies, and through the state. All of these employment arrangements often put Filipino caregivers in privatized residential care facilities for the elderly, assisted residential facilities, and private homes. This makes caregiving a prime precarious occupation because of its "hidden" nature, allowing for labor standards to be ignored while giving immigrants with various legal statuses an ability to work.[16] Finally, as an ethnic labor niche for Filipinos in the San Francisco Bay Area, eldercare consumers (whether at a residential care facility or one-on-one) have an expectation that there is an abundance of Filipino migrant workers in the area, which adds to the notion that they are disposable.

The sociocultural context of a privatized eldercare industry and a racialized and precarious workforce of Filipino migrants produces what I have called "normalized exploitation" for Filipina/o caregivers elsewhere.[17] In the context of Filipino caregivers' work conditions, I mark this concept to give readers a sense of how precarity shapes the lives of caregivers and the kinds of decisions they make in enduring work conditions that are clearly exploitative. I define this dynamic of "normalized exploitation" as caregivers accepting unfavorable working conditions because its "part of the job." For example, caregivers interpreted the nonstop nature of their work as "normal." From my grandmother Remedios's fourteen-hour days to care workers of the present, the tempo of a workday was not amenable to rest or meal breaks, especially when care workers have multiple clients.

Even for care workers who have one-on-one clients, they interpret their time "on the clock" as *bising-bisi*, or "back-to-back"—all of which is justified as part of the job.

Contrary to the California Domestic Workers Bill of Rights, which mandates ten minutes of uninterrupted break for every four hours of work, the quantitative portion of my study found that caregivers get an average minimum of twenty minutes of break time during a nine-hour workday. Way below the state mandate, that figure for care workers in our study is in an average of eight minutes of rest per four hours of work. Additionally, our study demonstrated that 64.5 percent of caregivers have their breaks interrupted, and 56 percent of caregivers have their sleep interrupted. Diana, one caregiver of two people per shift at a four-bed facility, responded to questions about her regular workday:

VALERIE: How many hours do you work in one day?
DIANA: 6 a.m. to 6 p.m. and I don't have a break. I end and it is nighttime already. In the morning, I wake up at 6 a.m. At the facility, I come up from my room in the basement, and I start cooking their food. After I finish cooking, I get their medicines ready. Then I set the table, make sure the food is on the table. Then at lunchtime I cook again, then dinnertime I cook again. They always have clothes that I wash, and I do that in between things so they all have clean clothes. When it's time for some of them coming home from their day, I start to clean up just before they get home. I help them get ready and shower for the evening. That's really most of my workday.
VALERIE: How about your lunchtime break?
DIANA: Food? A snack break? Ha ha! My lunch, if I get it, that is the only time I get to sit. I eat breakfast before anyone wakes up and at lunchtime, I eat standing up. That's it. There's no set break time for us.

Diana presents her workday in the interview as lacking a break. I vividly recall how my grandmother Remedios followed a schedule similar to Diana's twelve-hour day. The rapid way Diana lists her tasks marked by her cooking and the schedules of her clients at the residential care facility demonstrates that the pace of care workers is constant. Diana's scoff at the question about taking a break shows that even if care workers are mandated to take breaks, the reality of working with multiple clients and a limited staff means having a break between tasks is nearly impossible. While meal breaks are taken, Diana's description of "eating standing up" shows exactly what kind of respite she has during the day. Her acknowledgment that there isn't a set time for care workers to take a break normalizes this pace of work and the labor standards being broken at her workplace.

Che, a care worker in a six-bed residential care facility with three other care workers per shift, recounts her day, an echo of Diana's and Remedios's days:

CHE: Our routine starts with giving showers and helping bathe patients. Wake up and shower time right away.

VALERIE: Then?

CHE: Next, we prepare the breakfast! After shower we give breakfast, no? Right after, medication. And then medication . . . what else? Of course, we clean the house. Yes! After that we will clean the kitchen, after using the kitchen. Then the rooms, of course—after cooking and cleaning the kitchen. Mm-hm! We have, bed making, then continue the cleaning house. Uh! Toilet next! Bathroom and toilet scrubbing. They go in the living room or to the programs.

VALERIE: Then a little break time?

CHE: Oh, no breaks! When you wake up, straight to the 6 p.m. mark, until it's evening. Basically, twelve hours, right? Twelve hours straight, no break. No, no! No other choice, we should have to work back-to-back. What I mean to say is you don't have a choice. That's what we need to do because we need it [a wage] (rubs fingers together as a hand gesture for money). That's why we have to do it. That's the routine.

The workdays for Remedios, Diana, and Che display the tempo of a care worker's day in a residential care facility as nonstop and unrelenting. This is apparent. But at the end of Che's comment, she reminds us that her normalization of a twelve-hour day is, in fact, driven by her need for a wage. Che has two college-age children in the Philippines, and her top priority is to provide for their tuition and living expenses. The interwoven quality of her inability to take a break during the workday is partly an indication of the multiple tasks she is juggling as a care worker, and it is almost always in concert with her intrinsic motivation as a transnational mother. Scholars have established that the workdays of care workers in eldercare, child care, and as personal attendants is taxing given the multiple layers of domestic tasks they oversee.[18] The normalization of this exploitation is often justified by the types of financial assistance migrant care workers are committed to.

Elsewhere, Katherine Nasol and I have argued that this existing crisis for care workers has waned over decades, and the onset of the COVID-19 pandemic created a dual crisis for care workers' labor conditions.[19] Laura, a migrant mother who left a baby daughter in the Philippines in 1999, worked as a domestic worker in Taiwan and Saudi Arabia before coming to the United States. Upon arriving in the States in 2002, she immediately picked up work as a caregiver. Since then, her twenty-year tenure as a caregiver has provided her with lots of experience in working with a team of four care workers in a six-bed residential care facility and in a smaller care home with four beds. Her whole *kuwento* was anchored by her promise to give her daughter, Kim, the best future in terms of education and housing. She described her workday:

LAURA: Yeah, when we have six clients, then how many caregivers we have is dependent on our clients. Because the level 4Is have one-on-one. [Level 4I homes provide the highest level of services in a care facility.] They have support. So the one-on-one, from when they wake up, the licensing, they count those hours, there's an extra to the care provider. Then when they go to day program, that one that is like their school.

VALERIE: Yeah.

LAURA: Sometimes they pick them up at 7:30 a.m., 8:30 a.m., or 9 a.m., then they come back at 2 p.m., 2:30 p.m. or 3 o'clock. Then they count those hours again until they go to sleep for our wages.

VALERIE: Okay.

LAURA: Then that means there is four of us, and then our chores are bath, kitchen, beddings, and then the one, we call them floater, they rotate. At first it was a hard thing to learn, but the longer you do it, the easier it is to just keep working and working.

Laura describes this baseline of her work, which is similar to the others shared above. But during the COVID-19 pandemic, she remembers how the virus affected her work:

> The one that hurt the most, at least, we're all caregivers, and all our patients, we all became positive with COVID. We were just asymptomatic. No one got hospitalized, no one was on medicine, no 911, nothing. As in it was just us there, our boss kept us for fourteen days. Quarantined. We spent Christmas there. Sad but it's for your own good, and for the consumer. Yes, basically, I was the carrier. It was scary. Still the same, our life. It's still the same routine, but the addition was COVID, but it's the same routine. It devastated us, because imagine, every Saturday, we go out, we eat outside. You know, we go to McDonald's, Taco Bell, and everything. Then we go to the fairs, right? There's a state fair here. We go to—of course, because, it's like, you adapt them to the community. But then COVID happened, so you really can't go out anymore. It's just the same routine inside of the house. You get burnt out. You get burnt out. Especially when you were a stay-in and you can no longer leave. That is what is stressful.

This story of COVID transmission at Laura's six-bed residential care facility demonstrates the duality in the crisis of care workers in this industry. As a carrier of COVID-19, during the early parts of lockdown in 2020, not many care workers received information about the virus, given that details and studies on the virus were under way. And yet the normalized exploitation of their days continued, even during lockdown periods. Even during the times they contracted COVID, they were still expected to enact the same routines as described earlier. Without a secure avenue to paid sick leave, Laura and the four other care workers in the facility not only worked through the Christmas holiday, but they also continued to work while they were positive for the virus. In these examples, the dual crisis of "normalized exploitation" and COVID-19 produces conditions where care workers just continue to work despite illness. Laura's comment about thinking through her quarantine at work for the care workers' own good and the consumers' good seems logical to her because she had no other option of taking time off to nurse her health back to normal.

Still, while normalized exploitation is the backdrop of caregiver working conditions. I believe they continued to draw on practices and resources they had in their community to deal with the changing health crisis. During the beginning of the pandemic, I found there was a range of effects on caregivers' ability to continue to work. Stay-at-home orders meant that clients who needed part-time care during shorter periods of the day could hire only one or two attendants. However, live-in caregivers who worked at residential care facilities or assisted residential facilities were barely affected given that they were staying home at their workplace. Yet many used informal networks of resource sharing in the absence of formal information distribution to care workers in nonhospital settings to mitigate the "no work, no pay" reality of the pandemic. In a second PAWIS kuwentuhan, six Filipina caregivers, with ages ranging from their fifties to sixties, talked about the difference between caregiving before and during the pandemic:

CAROL: Umm, it's really hard because, you know, during this pandemic, you don't really know about anything of COVID. What is it? All we know is that [you] have to wear a lot of, you know, the PPE.

TERESA: Yes, you have to wear the PPE all the time. It's hard to adjust, it's hard to breathe because it's up to you, you need to protect yourself. Of course, before you don't have the thing on your face, so, yeah, it's very hard to get used to it, wearing it 24-7.

CAROL: And also, umm, you know, we, also fear for, for myself, also for my family, because I'm also a frontliner. Of course, so I need to protect myself for everyone here at the care home.

SHEILA: Yes, protecting yourself is important. So through PAWIS WhatsApp we just chat about what's the best mask if you are working with patients that are in and out of the clinic and doctor's appointment. Or where to get the gloves and how many—

TERESA: —How many times to sanitize your hands? (laughs) First you are learning how to do the oxygen tank, and now we are talking about how to stay out of the ER with COVID! Especially me, I'm easy to get flu!

In my research with caregivers, it was clear that many of them, just like the world over, were learning about the novel coronavirus as the pandemic spread in and across our communities, our cities, our nation, and the world. For caregivers, invisible frontliners, they were not privy to the same information as health-care workers in formal medical settings, so it was the same networks of information and resource sharing that assisted them in doing their jobs before the pandemic that stepped in to become hubs of information and practical advice that could be applied to their daily work.

TRANSNATIONAL LIVES, LOCAL DECISIONS

Past studies found that Filipinos do not identify their mental stressors as mental health issues until they have escalated into depression or suicide.[20] Filipino cultural values such as *tiis*, or a firmness in purpose, alongside Filipino familism, explain why caregivers underplay symptoms of mental health, since it puts primacy on their ability to support their families financially rather than recognizing initial feelings of stress and exhaustion. Therefore, while they may feel stressed, exhausted, and depressed as a result of their work conditions, Filipino caregivers may not label their symptoms as such given the sacrifice they are making for their families' well-being.

I draw attention to the transnational sociocultural contexts that govern how caregivers interpret their health and, consequently, their decisions to continue to work through mental and physical unwellness. Of the caregivers surveyed, 85.4 percent answered that they came to the United States for work employment and more work opportunities as means to improve their family. Serena, a caregiver with family in the Philippines, explains how her job benefits her family in the Philippines: "I have to move here. The salary is better here, right? Compared to ours [in the Philippines] . . . in dollars, you know. You know, like fifty is to one, so you would rather work here. Even your paycheck for one month here is equivalent to one year's worth of paycheck there [in the Philippines]." She went on to explain that her earnings in the United States converted to more Philippine pesos than if she were to work the same amount in any occupation in the Philippines. Like many caregivers in the study, Serena noted that her family depends on her monthly remittance for their daily sustenance. In fact, worrying about her family's ability to meet their basic needs is at the forefront of her mind daily. Serena's transnational and familial responsibility is the socio-contextual stress that has primacy over the workplace stress she experiences at her work. In this way, Serena's resolve (or "tiis") to deliver financial support drives her work ethic, despite the work conditions she may have as a caregiver. While the survey measured for symptoms of mental health stressors while at work, I can argue that Filipino caregivers' transnational contexts often induce stressors that may supersede the workplace factors they face daily. Without the proper contextualization of both transnational social relations with workplace conditions at residential care facilities, caregivers may interpret workplace stress as being secondary to their family obligations.

Utang ng loob, a cultural value that has been defined as social reciprocity, has been discussed as an obligation to return a favor, support, or service to a person in one's close circle.[21] In the context of the lives of migrant caregivers, one way this can manifest is in regular financial support. Many migrant caregivers interpret their financial support to the Philippines as a trade-off for not being physically present with their family members. The money they send home, then, is a way of meeting their filial debt while abroad, their reciprocity measured in capital rather than presence. For Filipino caregivers, utang ng loob under this specific sociocultural context is of great import as they negotiate their daily physical and mental health. Their ability to work every day regardless of health conditions describes not only their work ethic; in fact, it is anchored to their ability to provide for their families in the Philippines.

Richelle, a caregiver who left two school-age children in the Philippines eight years ago, now has two young adult children whom she hopes to go home to one day. In her kuwentuhan she recounts her experiences of exploitation and abuse from an employer who isolated her from any social circles outside of her work. Her current employer has been honest and transparent with her, which is why Richelle has stayed for eight years. Throughout her ordeal of being a caregiver abroad, she has been proud that her daughters have persisted in their education and graduated from both high school and college. In this way, Richelle feels guilt for missing so much of their lives, but she takes great pride in her ability to fund their education. Still, reuniting with her family is of great import. Richelle said:

> As long as I'm not with my kids, I should stay strong. I should have a goal, down the road: the ultimate goal is to be reunited with my kids and my mom. So that being established. Just, you know, acceptance of the situation. Stuff at work, I can handle. And I focus towards the goal of being reunited with my kids. So my mental health, I guess that's stable already, because of my goal.

In this quote Richelle demonstrates utang ng loob in identifying that her ultimate goal is to go home and be with her family, who have maximized her sacrifice of migration with graduating and finishing up their education. And although she has felt guilty for being away from her family, sending remittances to the Philippines is one way she shows her commitment to them. This necessarily means that Richelle would endure hard work situations and take on multiple jobs to be able to meet her family's needs. This utang ng loob, a debt Richelle feels toward her family, propels her work ethic.

Puri shared these sentiments about utang ng loob toward her family as well. When asked why she works so hard at her job, she responded, "For my family . . . in the Philippines. I still have a house that I am getting fixed, that's why. When the house gets finished, I'm going to lie low." This example of Puri's commitment to reciprocity to her family in the Philippines echoes Richelle's attitude about sending remittances to her family. Still, much of Puri's concern about improving her family's life in the Philippines disregards much of her own health outcomes as a caregiver in the Bay Area. After she reported that she never had a cold or flu in the eight years of being a caregiver, and that she only had back pain once as a result of her work, she later shared:

> Meron din paghirap sa pagiging caregiver. Araw araw, me diperensya sa sakit ng liko o kabalikat. Pero I'm okay, I'm fine. Sasabihin ko naman pag me isyu lang sa pamilya ko [in the Philippines]. Pag-ka ano naman, nagsasabi ako pag mahirap o hindi. Para kumampante naman sila doon.
>
> There are still difficulties in being a caregiver. Every day, there's a different pain in my back or shoulders. I will say something, though, if there's an issue with family [in the Philippines]. If there's something, I say something when I'm having a hard time or not. So they can calm down over there.

As I mentioned above in my comments about underreporting, Puri demonstrates the strong link between how she recognizes the pain in her body and leverages it to discipline her family in the Philippines. And while the intentions of her displaying her pain to her family is unclear, she shows that when she does feel her pain, it is precisely in the context of her transnational family.

The income of Filipino caregivers becomes a powerful way they stay connected to their families in the Philippines. And as they positively receive news of their families' various forms of stabilizing family life in the Philippines (e.g., graduation, housing, etc.), their work ethic and the spirit of "no work, no pay" is rewarded. In fact, the stressors at the workplace, especially exhaustion or workplace injury, become incidental to their view of their work as caregivers. When asked if she had the choice to either stay in the Philippines or move to the United States, Puri responded, "Right now I want to stay here because I'm working, and then, after that . . . I think I stay in the Philippines." Puri demonstrates that pressures of transnational obligations are attached to how she interprets her persistence as a caregiver.

CONCLUSION

Filipino caregivers do not see their transnational obligations simply as a burden. Rather, they see their jobs as caregivers as a privilege to maximize, in the name of their families in the Philippines. Without the sociocultural context of caregivers' Filipino cultural values such as tiis and utang ng loob, caregivers' underreported stress could be interpreted as an acceptance of their exploitative work conditions. However, the qualitative data and analysis indicate that when the survival of their family back home is dependent on migrant caregivers' income, the ability of caregivers to identify themselves as "stressed" is compromised. Furthermore, I argue that to identify themselves as stressed, caregivers would experience an impairment in their ability to care for their elderly patients and therefore disrupt their ability to support their families in the Philippines.

CHAPTER 2

INVISIBLE FRONTLINERS IN THE TIME OF CORONAVIRUS

In the fall of 2020, I held a Zoom *kuwentuhan* session in collaboration with PAWIS in Silicon Valley. Only a few months after the strict shelter-in-place lockdown in the state and across the United States, fifteen thousand Californians had already died from the virus, and the numbers were climbing rapidly. While hospitalizations remained dangerously high, essential workers not only continued to hold the front lines of hospitals, agriculture, food, and retail sectors but also provided care in various long-term facilities. In the evening Zoom meeting, I welcomed eight Filipina care workers joining from their live-in care facilities—from dining tables in common areas, to bedrooms with bunk beds in the background, to cleared kitchen counters of the residential care facilities for the elderly post-dinnertime.

The kuwentuhan session began with *kamustahan*—a lighthearted exchange of how people were feeling, what new *teleserye*, or series, one person was watching, and whether any of us had dinner yet since it was already eight o'clock. Three of the care workers were Zooming from their shared bedroom with one queen bed and a few armchairs. As they each shared their life updates, they passed an iPad around as they spoke, and other care workers would pop in from the side of the camera to tell a joke. This kuwentuhan session, unlike any I had facilitated before because of its Zoom platform, suddenly felt familiar. Although we were not exchanging Filipino food over a table and exchanging kamustahan over paper plates, all of us were at ease, people talking over one another, the highlighted "Speaker" picture switching as quickly as someone changed topics of discussion.

Soon enough, Tita Megan, a PAWIS worker leader, pivoted our chatter toward our session's topic: How has life changed with COVID-19? I began: "I wanted to ask everyone if there was a difference between working as a caregiver before COVID-19 and after the pandemic. What's the difference between working as a caregiver before the pandemic and after?" Together, Alicia, a sixty-year-old care worker in a care facility with four beds; Josie, a fifty-seven-year-old care worker across a few facilities; and Ellen, a sixty-five-year-old care worker with one patient, chimed in with their thoughts about the "difference":

ALICIA: Oh, yeah, it's a very big difference. It's really hard because, you know, during this pandemic, you have to wear a lot of, the PPE with you. It's hard to breathe because the mask is new, you need to protect yourself. Of course, unlike before, you don't have the thing on your face, so, yeah, it's very hard. And also, you know, we, I, also fear for myself, also for my family because I'm, also a frontliner. But no one tells me about the virus. So I need to protect myself for, for, for everyone here, my coworkers, my patients.

VALERIE: And what, what's the fear that you're feeling? Can you say a little more about what you felt afraid about?

ALICIA: I don't want to, of course, I don't want to get the virus from anyone. You know, I actually, I don't drive, so I used an Uber. Sometimes I take a bus. So I also have to meet up a lot of people there and you don't know anybody. Just anybody rides, in that car or that bus. You don't know what's going on with them or in there. Can you get the COVID there? So, yeah, I fear about that and if that happens . . . you'll have the, you know, virus. It's hard.

ELLEN: Yeah, so, it's about going to work. I mean, it's not just about work. It's about going to work, to being exposed in your, in your community, on your way. Is it on the bus seat? I just don't know much.

VALERIE: Were you ever nervous about working because caregiving is with people, with older folks, you know, the population that's most vulnerable? Did you ever feel worried about that?

SUSANNA: I am so worried about that because you don't, you don't really know. You don't know. Because anybody can be contracted by that virus. That's why I have to get myself checked. So I did have a COVID test. To make sure that I'm not contracted with anyone. So I'm happy about that. But then you're not sure again, because after that you will meet a lot of people again. So you don't know what's gonna happen. So it's not really calm. I try just protect myself, all the prevention, I do for myself. And for, for my family also.

JOSIE: I fear, you know, I'm worried that I will get the virus because you're dealing with so many people. I mean, the number of people know they come from so many different places. No one is telling us how the virus is working. So I have to protect myself and my husband because he is sick. Outside of work, I don't want to be meeting other people.

In this opening exchange among care workers, the level of uncertainty in their voices heightened. When each of them spoke about their fears, they held in tension the extrinsic motivations for their work—their family, their partners, the care workers in their facility, the patients they care for—as well as their fears for their own health and their multiple methods for prevention. What struck me as both a researcher and a person living during the pandemic, however, was the uncertainty under which the care workers operated. Their uncertainty was governed by a lack of information about the ever-changing virus, the lack of communication "down" the medical care ladder to home care workers doing the arduous, daily work of long-term care. And although at this point in the pandemic, government departments along with medical researchers were also just learning about the virus, care workers in this kuwentuhan session—and those across many similar conversations—worried that they would not get the right information to prevent the contraction and transmission of the virus in time.

In fact, studies on migrant worker psychosocial status during the COVID-19 lockdown demonstrated that many of them suffered from mental distress and anxiety regarding their jobs as care workers, especially in terms of housing and job insecurity.[1] The paradox of essential workers is that while various industries that consisted mostly of migrant workers in low-wage and precarious positions—namely, home health care, agriculture, retail, and food processing—were considered essential industries, the workers themselves were not deemed essential enough to be provided basic workplace protections and information about the virus.[2] As Alicia, Ellen, and Josie demonstrated in their conversation, much of their concern about the virus revolved around the same uncertainties that a majority of Americans were worried about. The major difference, though, was that they were putting themselves at risk daily for their jobs. In an unseen front line of the pandemic, care workers outside of hospital settings, in long-term care facilities, and in private homes in one-on-one care arrangements were last in line to receive information and protections from the COVID-19 virus.

While the American health-care system buckled under the strain of COVID-19, it continued its focus on acute care, patching holes on the capsizing hospital and care systems that tackled the rising COVID-19 hospitalizations. The lack of planning, and in fact the social imagination, for long-term and eldercare in the United States, relegated Filipina/o care workers who were staffing assisted living facilities, residential care facilities, and private homes to deeper invisibility. While the existing devaluation of care workers in this sector has been acknowledged by medical staff, doctors, and social workers alike, their important positions in the long-term care system remain precarious and low-wage. In short, the COVID-19 crisis compounded the standing crisis in long-term care in the United States. The experiences of Filipina/o care workers, from the reception of COVID-19 science and research to caring for themselves or their clients, to workplace protections such as sick leave or paid time off if they contracted the virus, shows that the maintenance of an underclass of care workers is vital to an American health-care system that exploits disposable ethnic immigrant care workers.

Scholars argue that during the pandemic, migrant care workers had to choose between safeguarding their health or losing their job(s), to the detriment of the family members that relied on their financial support.[3] Migrant care workers were caught in multiple interlocking systems of domination that rely on their identities as migrants (undocumented or otherwise), women, people of color, transnational breadwinners, and precarious laborers. Their experiences as care workers under COVID-19 have been shaped by the systems that refuse to valorize their work as essential and put them at a disadvantage as immigrants, women, and people of color working in uncertain industries. During the rise of COVID in 2020, anti-Asian racism led people to target Filipino and Asian ethnic migrant care workers.[4] As I will show, racism became a decisive interlocutor in the work conditions of Filipina/o care workers. I argue that these systematic constraints affect Filipino care workers' abilities to demand fair work conditions and insist on labor standards in their workplaces.

In this chapter, I discuss in depth the experiences of Filipina/o care workers working during the COVID-19 pandemic. Specifically, it is important to note that the qualitative data I include was collected during shelter-in-place orders in Bay Area, California, counties starting in March 2020 and continuing after the date when the orders were lifted in June 2020 and through the fall of 2020. Thus the insights in this chapter reflect the early parts of the COVID-19 pandemic, when care workers' lives were in major and continual transition. In the following pages, I describe their workplaces as an "invisible front line" because Filipina/o care workers in this study worked with the most vulnerable population for COVID-19 contraction and death—those sixty-five years old and older with preexisting health conditions—thus making these care workers most susceptible to contraction and illness. While their work on the front line was essential, the work conditions, the risk in working their jobs without basic protections, and the logic under which they continued to put their health on the line have yet to be explored in a sociological mode. I argue that caregiving during the pandemic exacerbated the crises of their work and impacts on their health, as I discussed in the last chapter. For Filipinos, caregiving at this hazardous time was working under a dual crisis in the long-term care industry. Moreover, I establish that the transnational sociocultural contexts of their lives made it even more difficult for them to assert their rights to workplace protections or advocate for themselves.

UNCERTAIN TIMES, CERTAIN RISKS

Ian, a forty-four-year-old migrant father of two children in the Philippines, was a trained nurse in the Philippines. Although his credentials did not migrate with him—his formal training is not commensurate with his current job and salary—he knew he could apply his medical expertise in the caregiving industry in the Bay Area. Before the pandemic, Ian worked part-time as a certified nurse assistant (CNA) at an assisted living facility with seventy-five beds, and he also picked up shifts on his days off or after early shifts at a smaller residential care facility. I had a socially distanced conversation with him in the backyard of the four-bed facility where he worked four months after shelter-in-place orders were lifted. His comments demonstrated the shifting conditions under which he, and many like him, took risks during the onset of COVID-19 pandemic. Ian said:

> It's a lot more difficult now. First of all, because there's that fear of uncertainty. You don't know what the case will be or what the setup will look like. Not just for me but in general, caregivers today are careful with the patients that they work with. As much as possible, [they] stay away from facilities because there will be a lot of people. Second, if the patient has had COVID in the past, of course that's scary because I wouldn't want to catch COVID and spread it to other people. There's a lot to consider today because of the situation. Some caregivers now aren't working because of fear; most of them don't have private cars so they have to commute, and the concern will always be there. Third, how much is the rate today? If it's okay or if it's the same. I think there's not as much people taking up caregiving right now. Are they in demand? Or is the salary low? Or I don't know if there might be a lot more people taking up caregiving right now because of the COVID situation? But your family in the Philippines doesn't go away. They still need you to send money. The economic situation is worse there!

Step by step, Ian explained the costs and benefits of working as a caregiver in the Bay Area while vaccines for the pandemic were still in development. To work from Ian's concept of concerns under COVID, in this next section I expound on the three themes that he highlighted: (1) the availability of care work in the pandemic and its impacts on the livelihood of Filipinos; (2) the kinds of risks and choices Filipino care workers had to make working on the front lines, from their commutes, to considerations about the people they lived with, to workplace protections or the lack thereof; and (3) the role of family—transnational and local—in how Filipina/o migrants navigated working in the care industry during the pandemic. I share evidence about how the precarity in the industry of caregiving was magnified.

Shifts in Work and Wages

When asked on my survey, "How did the COVID-19 pandemic affect your work hours?," Filipino care workers reported that schedules became more volatile, with shifts sometimes increasing and sometimes decreasing. During kuwentuhan we explored these answers in greater depth to parse the important details that separate full-time and part-time care workers. Some live in their facilities and work full-time. Many others, especially the most vulnerable, are "live-out" workers—they patch together a quilt of various part-time caregiving jobs between small and large facilities, one-on-one care arrangements, and jobs in other industries like retail or restaurants. The pandemic either intensified full-time, live-in care work or destabilized the ability of part-time workers to access their patchwork employment.

For the first group of full-time, live-in care workers, shelter-in-place orders and the vulnerability of their clients kept them cordoned off from the world. Rowena, a full-time, live-in care worker who has worked at a residential care facility, said, "Nothing much changed, not much—at least not with the caregivers working in a care facility—because nothing changed. Like specifically in our care home we had an early lockdown. So nobody comes in. No outsider comes in. And then we have put precautionary measures [in] right away, even before the state declares a total lockdown. They need us to stay here, so while others were losing jobs, we'll always have jobs. Because we just stay here."

Lorraine, a full-time, live-in care worker in a five-bed residential facility, elaborated:

> The number of hours, it increased more. Supposed to be eight hours only, now its twelve hours. Because there are only three live-in. And we usually have a fourth live-out. But they cannot come inside. So in some way I'm happy because my paycheck is bigger now. Yes, so that means I can make

> more money. But it's also hard because, for example, in the beginning for the masks. Only four piece[s] per person. Then when you're done with the four you have to disinfect it and dry it out. I said, "Why is it like that?" They don't give us PPE! We have to disinfect? And dry it out? Gloves like that too. Oh my god! Even if we used it for a long time, they make us reuse it. There are two or three of us caregivers and we have to share all the gloves, oh my god! I request and they said no because it was out of stock.

In Lorraine's account of her work hours increasing, she traced the change as a welcome difference in her paycheck, and then quickly she remembered the risk and panic she felt in her job given that the PPE was not provided to the workers in her facility. In many ways, live-in care workers like Lorraine had to work more hours during lockdowns and time periods where in-and-out privileges were constrained. But often that change in their biweekly paycheck also translated to intensified work inside the facility. Whether that meant they could not or would not take breaks during the workday, or that they were literally locked down in their workplace because it was also where they lived, the working conditions—coupled with fear and panic from the pandemic—intensified their day-to-day tasks.

Another caregiver, Richelle, worked full-time in a care home but lived outside of the facility. Unlike her other colleagues, Richelle described what happened during lockdown as the "world was closing in":

> Yeah, that. Our hours were increased, things like that. That's okay. But COVID devastated us in a different way—imagine, every Saturday we go out. We eat outside. You know, we go to McDonald's, Taco Bell, and everything. Then we go to the fairs, right. There's a state fair here. Then we go to Cinco de Mayo. We go to these outside events, of course, because, it's like you adapt them to the community. So we go to the Pumpkin Festival, whatever, things like that. But now we can't do that anymore because we have two patients that are easily sick. Then COVID happened, so you really can't go out. It's sad for the clients. But it's hard for us too. No, we can't go out anymore. It's hard on our hearts and our minds too.

If they are able, care workers create opportunities for their clients to get out in the world. The advantages of this are numerous for clients, but it's also good for care workers to see the community events around them and be outside of the care facility where they work and live. Lorraine's last sentiment about the hardship on care workers' "hearts and minds" blew me away. Although a trip to McDonald's on Saturday may seem trivial, it is a chance for workers and clients to have a change of scenery and experience something different from their day-to-day schedules. While this example does not connote an intensified work condition in terms of daily tasks, it points to a different type of intensity—the rote and repetitive schedule of live-in caregivers. Under COVID, with limited mobility concerning their clients' health and safety, as well as their own, care workers had no reprieve from their full-time work.

For the second group of care workers, their access to part-time work increasingly became limited because of the pandemic restrictions on exposure and social interactions. Before the pandemic, part-time care workers secured their "gigs" in two ways: either affiliating with an employment agency or receiving referrals through informal networks among care workers. On the one hand, agencies coordinate care services for clients who might need assistance with their daily living activities for part of a day or only several days a week. Therefore care workers are able to request certain days and can be assigned work when they need it. This flexibility is what many care workers find positive. Care workers agree to an hourly wage that can hover under or a bit over minimum wage, based on a person's experience, although there is a monthly fee that care workers have to pay to the agency. Care workers have reported that their relationships with agencies can sour because a worker's "cut" gets squeezed, especially in unstable part-time work. On the other hand, finding work among informal immigrant networks through church fellowships or community organizations can bring opportunities that are stable and not tied to a third party. However, in these connections, Filipino cultural value can obligate workers to their immigrant friends and acquaintances. These ties can set up care workers to endure exploitation and abuse in the workplaces they are connected to. Both of these methods to secure part-time work are often complemented by work in retail stores, nearby gas stations, or in the restaurant industry as cashiers or cooks. During the pandemic, these tenuous connections became even more unstable. It also made it more difficult for care workers to achieve the hours they worked before state policies severely constrained interactions and mobility.

Lia, a forty-four-year-old care worker who also works at a Target store part-time, reflected on picking up part-time shifts from her employment agency: "I am always getting canceled—like, let's say I'll pick up shifts, but in COVID there are still a higher chance that I'll get canceled. Like, let's say I'll put in fifteen shifts on . . . the days I can work. I can work these fifteen days. Out of that fifteen days in one month, they'll probably just gonna give me or let me work ten—ten of those fifteen shifts that I asked for." In the past, the ability to work fifteen days out of a month as a care worker alongside her part-job at Target helps her receive a paycheck that can support her basic needs in the United States and to remit to her family in the Philippines. Under COVID-19, her monthly paycheck was severely affected by her inability to be assigned part-time work through her agency.

Like Lia, Linda, a care worker with a twenty-five-year career in the caregiving industry, also reported that COVID-19 had deleterious effects on her monthly bottom line. I asked, "Has COVID affected your work?" Linda retorted, "Absolutely! (laughs) So I usually work twelve hours a day for, like, three days a week. And I'm okay with that. Twelve hours a day. It's okay, I can survive it. But now for COVID, it was, like, eight hours a day, for four days. I'm just barely making it. I cannot go to two, three part-times. I have to only stay in one for one day." When I inquired about how it affects Linda's ability to pay her bills every month, she said, "Well, I'm trying to save some money when I can put some in my savings. But you know if it's not enough, I have to get more money from the savings and put it to pay my rent." Both Lia and Linda demonstrate that while part-time work allowed them flexibility before the pandemic, during the pandemic the lack of access to part-time work affected their ability to sustain themselves.

Workplace Exposures and Risks

Many care workers described working during the pandemic as *nakakastress*, or stressful. They gave multiple reasons, spanning the lack of information about COVID-19 to their anxieties about contracting the virus and exposing themselves inadvertently to it. Much of their stressors were produced because care workers on the front lines of long-term care were not afforded similar protections and public information about the virus. Rina said, "There is a risk when you are on public transportation, on the bus, on the BART train. Because I didn't know much about COVID-19, there's a risk that I don't want to take a chance that I will bring the germs to the facility." While the lack of information and understanding about the virus shaped how care workers chose to commute to their jobs, it also guided their decisions to stop working.

Rosselle, a fifty-year-old care worker with diabetes and a history of respiratory illness, explained the risks she faced working during the pandemic:

> *Kase* because of the COVID. I don't want to work as much. Before, five days I would work at [a] facility as a caregiver. The facility has one hundred beds. In that facility, there will be so many staff, so many nurses, so many patients. So too much people. So I quit there. And then in another city, I work at the rehab. So I stopped working my two days on. There I was hourly. Sometimes eight hours. Sometime[s] twelve hours. But I have to commute from here, so there is a risk when I am on public transportation, right? Bus. BART train. Bus. There's a risk that . . . I don't want to take. So I quit that. I don't want to take chance *kase* because I am working three days in a private home. And of course, the patient is elderly, I might bring germs to him, through my breathing or during my eating lunch? That's why I quit the facility. That's why I just stay home and then the private one-on-one work.

Rosselle did not receive the quickly changing information about the virus—whether it was transmissible via droplets, as it was first publicly reported, or if it was airborne.

More important, as part-time care workers without standardized labor protections like paid sick leave or medical benefits, much of the cost-benefit analysis for care workers relied on if they could show up to work the next day. If commuting on a bus or train would expose them to the virus and they became sick, the risk would be too high to take. If working at a large facility that exposed them to a large number of staff and patients, which in turn could put them at risk of contraction, then care workers erred on the side of caution. Especially for part-time workers like Rosselle, a chief concern for workers was transmitting the virus to their one-on-one patients who were most vulnerable to contracting and dying from COVID-19. Rosselle continued: "Well, I have issues with my lungs before, right? I'm hospitalized with it. So during COVID, I could not even think of my own health. If I got the COVID, will it be worse off for me?" Care workers had to weigh their decisions to work by choosing between looking out for their own health and their preexisting conditions, their exposure in transit or at their workplaces and transmitting to their clients. Given that caregivers have been continually denied basic labor rights, such as paid sick leave, risking getting sick with COVID was simply a hazard many of them had to live with.

For many caregivers I interviewed in the midst of the pandemic, many reported mental health stressors that I interpret as issues of fear and panic, anxiety and isolation. Early on, so much of the virus and caring for those who might get sick or who were already sick with it was unclear and disconcerting for Filipina caregivers. In a kuwentuhan with caregivers who were members of PAWIS, Irma described the fear and panic she felt when news of the pandemic started to hit mainstream media. Just a few months before shelter-in-place orders were mandated, the caregivers in her facility were calling in sick:

> The word COVID wasn't popularized yet because it was in January (2020). I was wondering why things were the way they were at work. Everyone at work was getting sick and then calling in absent, and why were they taking so long to recover? Then they would get better, or even if they weren't better, they'd still go to work. Then people started to gargle with warm water and salt. "Drink vinegar," they said. When the news of COVID cropped up, I said, "Was that what happened to us? Was that COVID or not? Because it wasn't just me that was sick; it was all of us. But can we get it again? Is there something wrong with us? Should we keep working?"

Irma was astute about the shift in how she and her coworkers were getting sick before the pronouncements of the pandemic were validated in the media and public health mandates. However, her mind was filled with unanswered questions that led to self-doubt about her ability to care for herself while being in a healthy environment to work with others and care for their clients.

In my final series of questions for Irma, her train of thought stitched together her hesitation about her own health and the long-term effects of COVID and her efficacy as a caregiver. Although Irma discussed later on that she did not stop working through shelter-in-place, mostly because many of her coworkers were falling ill with the virus, scholars have argued that the workload of health-care workers increased dramatically because of additional duties due to client care complications and the growing number of colleagues taking sick leave.[5] While studies demonstrated that the mental health of health-care workers in hospital settings suffered greatly due to similar work conditions, there has been little discussion about the impacts on care workers in long-term care in facilities like the one Irma worked in.[6] In fact, Vanessa Banta and Geraldine Pratt have argued that the geographies of the private home or privatized care facilities were just out of the sight of the American public eye and the regulation of the buckling American health-care system under crisis. Therefore the COVID-19 crisis "led to an intensification of (im)mobilities for many categories of essential workers" that entrapped many caregivers at the workplaces.[7]

Other workers in my research reported increased stress based on their efficacy as caregivers. Justine, a fifty-five-year-old caregiver, reflected on adjusting to new protocols with her client:

> And I was doing, um, a lot more than I felt qualified for. And because no one's trained me on that. And then she had IV antibiotics, um, that she was given through a pump, and I've never done that. They quickly trained me at the hospital, but I was so nervous about it. And I had to do that every day for six weeks. So that was—I felt like someone should have been paying me somehow, but because I wasn't doing something I was comfortable with, and it was something I worried about all the time. So, yeah, I wish maybe there was also a medical training or something for caregivers or something in addition to compensation just to relieve anxiety.

During the kuwentuhan, I could hear Justine's anxiety ratchet up by the way she blurted out all of her worries and then her proposed resolution so quickly. Justine's fast-paced response to my question about the changes in her workplace signaled that the stressors at work took a toll on how she perceived herself as an effective caregiver, especially as new information about COVID-19 added to her workload. With or without training, Justine still attended to the needs of her clients. On this invisible front line, the addition to Justine and Irma's workloads and shifts was without additional recognition or remuneration. Justine continued: "I felt like I was here. I was there. I had new things to do. And all in the same amount of hours and the same amount of pay." For Justine and many caregivers, their wages are of great import to their own survival and to their families' financial health. However, during COVID, with the relentless changes in work duties and shifts, caregivers' worried that they couldn't keep up with providing quality care—and that concern was often on par with their concerns about not being paid enough for their increased workload. I think it is important to note that the paramount issue to caregivers during COVID was being able to provide quality health care to their clients.

Long-term care facilities, especially for the elderly who survived the pandemic in its early phases, when the vaccines had not yet been developed, were such an important site for understanding how the virus affects people after recovery. For all intents and purposes, the residential care facilities and assisted residential facilities were front lines that were not properly acknowledged in our popular imagination but, more practically, for access to the incessantly updating health facts on COVID. While the expectations for caregivers were high, employers, such as elderly clients and families of those clients, did not understand that caregivers were not part of the larger health-care chain. They did not receive timely training and additional information about caring for surviving clients, outside of medical professionals' advice for individual clients. While clients became frustrated with caregivers because they were not up to speed about COVID care, many caregivers suffered as invisible frontliners. For example, Linda, a sixty-year-old caregiver, lamented the experiences that were affecting her mental state working one-on-one with a client. Through tears she said:

> I get, like, upset sometimes. So it's, like, I just wanted to just quit or something. Actually I give up one client, because I just couldn't take it anymore. They keep asking me why I don't know anything about COVID.

> They, you know, they abuse me—They know that they can do anything to us ... the way they treated their caregivers as like [because] they're paying a lot of money for our work and therefore that they wanted to get their money's worth. So they are talking to you like you don't know anything. You're not a nurse. You're just a caregiver. It makes me feel so low. They make you feel like you're nothing.

In this comment, Linda expresses that the treatment she received and the berating she underwent with one of her clients led her to feeling unworthy and undervalued. Caregivers' position as invisible frontliners was so clear to me when Linda said she was being criticized for not knowing anything about COVID. When the existing disparities in the health-care systems and in public health institutions faced the COVID crisis, the hardest hit were patients and care workers. The inequitable distribution of resources across health sectors produced experiences of disempowerment and marginalization.[8] The burden that Linda felt was the de-professionalization of caregiving coupled with a lack of understanding by consumers about how disjointed the health-care sectors are. For Linda, a part of her depression was about her employers' constant criticism, but it was also because providing care for her elderly client was a job she took seriously. Debating on continuing with this client, Linda had a heavy burden to carry around just how much she could take living the contradiction of failing systems, irate employers and the invisible front line.

For some care workers, the risk of taking public transportation was too high. Sherry recounted, "During the early time of the pandemic, I didn't have my own car. But I don't think going to the bus was a good idea. What if I got COVID on my way to work? So I just call Uber or Lyft. Before I enter the care homes that I part-timed at, I really had to sanitize my hands because I know that I was in an Uber. And my coworkers would say right when I'm at the door, 'Did you sanitize?'" And although this risk-reducing practice ensured that care workers would limit their interactions with the public, hiring a private car to get to work also cost them money out of pocket, for which employers did not reimburse them. Sherry continued: "Uber was expensive in the pandemic. It cut into my check. A lot. I didn't get sick then, so I guess it was worth it. But it was expensive to get to work safely." Mitigating these risks to exposure had their obvious benefits, but care workers also incurred unexpected economic costs.

Additionally, many care workers themselves are aging migrants with preexisting health conditions. Jenni, a fifty-six-year-old care worker and diabetic, said, "I have been a diabetic way back in the Philippines. And I have been diagnosed with ulcers since May 2016. Since May 2016 I have chronic disability so these are issues I think of. Will I get the virus? Will I recover?" Many care workers weigh their own health as less important than their ability to do their job on a day-to-day basis. Because most care workers are afforded neither medical benefits nor access to regular health care by private employers or employment agencies, care workers do not care to miss work because of their financial need. While the 1938 Fair Labor Standards Act (FLSA) legislated basic labor rights for many workers, domestic workers—a majority of whom were Black American women—were explicitly drawn out of these workplace protections.[9] To this day, the FLSA continues its racialized and gendered legacy by excluding Filipina care workers, among other domestic workers in the United States. The intertwined historicity of racial and gendered domestic labor exclusions increased the possibility of health inequities for Filipina/o care workers under COVID-19. The covert and systemic racism that had removed care workers' ability to choose their own well-being over making a wage was then exacerbated by the overt racism they experienced on the job during the pandemic.

While care workers picked up what part-time shifts they could get during the pandemic, they were not just concerned about their exposure to the virus on their commutes to work or in their workplace. Amid the pandemic, the blatantly racist narratives that spread from the seat of power in the United States, notably from then president Donald Trump, contributed to the uptick of anti-Asian racism. A through line in Asian American history, prejudiced and misinformed publics blamed the pandemic on Asian immigrants and Asian Americans, attributing Asian bodies as carriers of disease.[10] While the racialized discourse of "yellow peril" is a vestige of white supremacist and racist ideologies against growing Asian powers and Asian immigration to the United States, Filipina/o care workers in the contemporary moment felt the brunt of these nativist and racist tropes.

Part-time care workers in the pandemic were often sent out to their assignments based on their availability and the need of clients for in-home care.

During a kuwentuhan session, Roanna, a fifty-two-year-old caregiver who has always worked part-time because she enjoys meeting new clients and has her own car, described an interaction that made her pause: "I think it was June of 2020, lockdown just got done. The agency gave me a client. And I go to the house, with a cheery mood. I'm always cheery. The white couple who I was supposed to assist stop me at the front door. 'Are you Asian?' 'Oh, no you don't have to come here,' he said. 'Don't come here!' So I turned around and I left."

After Roanna recalled this story, she paused for a few minutes, choking back tears. Another caregiver, Felicia, jumped in to comfort her: "We are not Filipino when we go to work. We are Asian now. And they think COVID is our fault."

Other care workers in this kuwentuhan session shared how scared they felt because the concept of the "China virus" might make employers turn them away at the door or cease their contracts. In an effort to recover their dignity, many of them reminded one another of the work ethic of Filipino care workers, stepping in to work in an industry that has been abandoned. They were making sense of the racist interactions they have had with employers and the public through their worth as workers who continually show up to care for their clients. Felicia's comment about becoming "Asian" in the pandemic struck me as an important moment of racial consciousness among the care workers in the kuwentuhan. As they affirmed one another's work ethic, their dialogue about the fear of being Asian during the pandemic came through strongly because of the anti-Asian narratives that surrounded them, from the president's frequent derogatory remarks to the rapid increase in anti-Asian interpersonal violence during the early part of the pandemic.

In another instance, I interviewed Grace, a fifty-five-year-old care worker who had been working in the caregiving industry for fifteen years. Grace had worked in live-in facilities and was taking up part-time care work to financially contribute to her daughter as she finished college. In a tearful exchange over Zoom in the summer of 2020, just after the shelter-in-place orders were lifted, Grace explained an interaction with a new white American client to whom her employment agency had assigned her. When Grace arrived to start a part-time job caring for an elderly white woman for three mornings each week, the client's daughter, a white woman, acquainted Grace with her mother's routine:

GRACE: And they [employers] were saying to each other that, "Oh, all the caregivers are Filipino?" and I said, "Well, Filipinos like to work as a caregiver and we have the passion to help, you know, the elderly and do you expect the other race to work with you?" And then they didn't say anything, but they talked loudly that Filipinos are taking all the jobs as a caregiver. But the fact of the matter is, nobody wants to work as a caregiver.

VALERIE: And did they have another preference? You, you, you feel like they wanted someone else, not a Filipino?

GRACE: Yes, I think they wanted like to say . . . a Caucasian or something. Yeah, because they don't like the Black people too. They don't like Black caregivers.

VALERIE: How do you know?

GRACE: They said that they don't like Filipino. They don't like Black caregivers. They don't like Filipino. So I go.

As Grace wiped away her tears—and I wiped mine away too—I told her that the treatment she received was wrong. She responded by telling me about her decade-and-a-half-long experience with so many white clients, Black and Asian clients, whom she nursed back to health, whose life stories she listened to, whose lives she enriched. She was confounded as to why this woman and her daughter had discriminated against her.

Grace never went back to that client. She chalked up the event to the "COVID situation," and when I asked what she meant by "situation," she answered simply, "It's the virus. Americans think Filipinos and Asians are the virus too." In this response, Grace linked how the virus and "America," the nation's narrative around COVID-19, was one way to explain why she received the racist, anti-Asian treatment at the hands of her client. Her explanation conflating "virus" and Asianness demonstrates that Grace understood that her clients' racialization of her was a reason why she was refused work that day. Sociologist Miliann Kang has argued that contestations over Asian migrant workers' bodies, especially in service and domestic work industries, reflect long-standing divisions around race, immigration, and gender.[11] In fact, the macro-level narratives shape the ways Asian migrant workers manage the emotional labor in their highly physically taxing jobs. In the midst of a racist interaction, Filipino caregivers must manage their emotions, the emotional context of their employers, and, during the COVID-19 pandemic, suffer financially from racist narratives that are read onto the bodies of caregivers.

Many caregivers lost work and wages because of blatant prejudice and racist discrimination, Tracy, a caregiver in her late forties who works as a part-time caregiver while juggling her own dialysis, recounted a time when she felt that a job had been taken away because of her early contraction of COVID-19 and the conflation of the virus with Asian communities in the United States:

> I was working one-on-one in February, before the COVID. But I felt sick, sore throat and my nasal congestion worsened, I couldn't breathe. I had fever. So I took Sudafed. I just bought at the pharmacy, the Sudafed, until the sickness went away. Yeah, I think it was the COVID. It was three weeks. While I was so sick at home, I told the agency, "I can't work right now." So I didn't have money, nothing to pay rent, nothing. I didn't work, then I got better. I wanted to go back to work. But my client said, "Oh, no, you don't have to come here," she said, then she gave me $150 and said, "Don't come here anymore because we know you got sick, and it's the Asians getting people sick." So then I have to go back to the agency to get a different work. The agency didn't do anything.

Before I analyze this quote, I note the lack of labor protections for caregivers, wherein Tracy had no health insurance to visit a doctor, her only recourse was an over-the-counter medicine, Sudafed. She did not have paid sick leave to be able to care for herself when she was sick with COVID, and therefore the weeks that she was sick meant she would have no income and would not be guaranteed work when she was well enough.

Considering that Tracy had preexisting conditions when she had symptoms of COVID-19, I was saddened to hear that she went through such a health crisis on her own. In her retelling of her story, Tracy moved pretty quickly away from discussing being turned away by her client due to her race. Her concern, rightfully so, was to secure another job since she was sick for so long. Still, it adds to the evidence that anti-Asian racism permeated the ability of caregivers to obtain work. However, I point to employment agencies and their lack of accountability to provide reliable information to their clients about the transmission of the COVID virus, which has nothing to do with a caregiver's racial background. While public health professionals have recommended that direct measures be communicated to clients and employers of care workers, the long-term care industry, which exists without centralized systems of information dissemination and communication, failed to protect workers and create work conditions free from racist discrimination.[12] Quite the opposite, the neoliberal governance of care not only allowed for this type of racial aggression, but I argue that it is part of the way long-term care operates.

Sheila, an immigrant and caregiver in her late fifties who has worked in the industry for a decade or more, talked about the racist turn in her experience working with one-on-one clients during the pandemic: "After the COVID, you need to have patience because sometimes they get on your nerves. The patient and the family, they don't listen to you and [are] demanding. Sometimes they verbally abuse you, they say, 'Why are you here?!' 'COVID comes from China!' Like that. A lot of verbal abuse because they're demanding a different worker." The increase of racist and white supremacist discourses that racialized the COVID-19 contagion as inherently Chinese and, therefore, Asian, illustrates that the danger and violence of such tropes were manifold. During this discussion in our kuwentuhan, Sheila was shaking her head about the treatment she received from one of her clients and the verbal abuse she sustained working there. Her comment about the need to have patience was a kindness that she extended to that client and the family. Thus, I present her story and apply Philippine studies scholar Jean de Borja's concept of "emotional labor of persistence" to the situation to demonstrate the emotional labor and vulnerability of care workers whose workplaces are precarious in that they work in private homes without protection.[13] Along with the risk of contracting and transmitting the virus, many care workers managed the emotional labor of appeasing their employers in their workplaces, although the overt racial discrimination took work and wages away from them, diminishing their purpose and dignity as care workers. Some also described the fear of being in public at the cost of being read as Asian. With the uncertainties of their jobs, the sociopolitical contexts of anti-Asian racism mar the experience of caring under COVID-19.

COVID-19 IN THE TRANSNATIONAL FAMILY

The COVID-19 pandemic was and is a global experience. For Filipinos in the United States and the Philippines, and arguably the diaspora, the simultaneous navigation through shelter-in-place and an indefinite future varied with location, but it remained a unique moment in the lives of families separated over extended periods of time and long distances. For these economic and social reasons, the pandemic provided a semblance of going through a common experience together—93 percent of Filipina/o migrants who participated in my study during the pandemic had been immigrants for more than five years. Many of them had used multiple types of information and communication technologies (ICTs) such as Facebook, Instagram, WhatsApp, Viber, and FaceTime to build relationships across borders for years. Digital connectivity as a practice of family making has been a characteristic of transnational Filipino families for decades.[14] The digital intimacies across transnational Filipino families facilitate routine domestic labor and practical matters in households, including care for children, cooking meals, and cleaning tasks. The communication that transnational Filipino family members practice also manage the emotions, tensions, and conflicts that emerge. These family-making and intimacy-building practices among migrants and their families allowed many people to remain in communication through the early parts of the pandemic and continue through today's pervasive conditions. While other non-migrant families were adjusting to keeping in touch via screens, transnational Filipino families relied on the same ICTs and behaviors they had relied on in the past. The only difference was that enforced separation and digital connectivity were now the conditions that everyone lived in under COVID-19.

While families were sharing day-to-day information regarding the unfolding of COVID-19 in their own locations, Filipina/o care workers in the Bay Area were even more concerned about their families in the Philippines.

The impacts of a halted economy in a developing nation like the Philippines were felt significantly with the loss of livelihood for Filipinos whose work was contractualized and deemed nonessential. In industries like business process outsourcing, otherwise known as "call centers," where a majority of young educated Filipinos work, the lockdown effectively froze the industry for months.[15] Scholars have argued that the loss of jobs reverberated across the Filipino labor diaspora. Labor migrants who were land- and sea-based were repatriated to the Philippines in droves.[16] Migrants' repatriation was a blow to that country's economy, which is reliant on the remittances of labor migrations worldwide. While the economic health of the country was suffering, moreover, Filipina/o care workers who were in constant communication with family members in the Philippines and other countries were even more convinced that migrants working abroad must do their best to stay healthy and work through the pandemic.

In a kuwentuhan session at the latter part of shelter-in-place, four Filipina care workers discussed the fear of contracting COVID-19. Joanna and Kristine, both live-in caregivers at the same facility, participated via the same Zoom screen, and Cynthia and Mari, both part-time care workers, each joined from their own homes. Our jovial discussion dipped in and out of seriousness and laughter:

JOANNA: I said, Where will I quarantine? What am I gonna do? What's gonna happen to me? I just pray, "Lord *tulungan mo ko* . . . help me! I hope I don't get sick!" (laughs)

CYNTHIA: I hope I don't get sick. I don't have cough. But I also don't have tonsils anymore. Will I be protected? I still gargle with saltwater, I'm so paranoid. I hope I don't get sick.

KRISTINE: *Talagang napaparanoid ka*, of course you'll be paranoid! What will happen to you? What will happen to your family in the Philippines? Hungry! That's what! (laughs)

JOANNA: What will happen to us? What? We can't go back to the Philippines! When I talk to them on Messenger, I see no work there. We're all going to shrivel up and die together, even without COVID! (laughs)

MARI: Of course, no. They rely on us! They rely on us *na hindi magka-COVID*, to not get COVID! We're all in this mess together, but the difference is I have to work. I have to send money. I have to keep sending. We all experience and scared of COVID, but for me, I cannot be scared.

In kuwentuhan the jest always echoes truth. The exchange above drew a through line between care workers' concerns about contracting COVID-19, the practical questions about how to deal with the virus, and importantly, how their health status in the United States will affect many in the Philippines. I have written elsewhere about how Filipina migrants working in New York City make everyday decisions based on their families' well-being in the Philippines and sometimes vice versa.[17] In a city across the United States, San Francisco, in a different social and political moment, one constant is Filipina/o migrants' transnational families as a core node for decision-making processes in everyday life. More than worrying if an illness or virus may cause grave consequences like death, the foremost concern for Filipina/o care workers is the welfare of their families in the Philippines. The simultaneity of experiencing a global pandemic was acknowledged by the workers, however, as Mari referred to her family's reliance on her as not being solely the monthly remittance she sends. Mari's family is banking on the promise that she can stay healthy and continue in her work.

Cherry, a migrant mother of two young daughters in the Philippines and a care worker in a residential care facility with five beds, talked about her experience of mothering in the pandemic as *nakakaloka*, or crazy-making: "I'm worried if they're gonna get COVID. If I'm gonna get COVID. Thank God that my parents are caring for them. I want to go back to them, but what's important is that I keep working, right? And that they are okay there in Pinas." In the order of things in Cherry's mind, her children contracting COVID-19 is primary in how she formulates the logic of continuing on to work. She continued: "I talk to them on [Facebook] Messenger and FaceTime all the time. I try to keep in contact, even at work. Since we're all inside anyway, why not?" One way that Cherry deals with the "crazy-making" conditions of living, working as a care worker, and transnational mothering in the pandemic is the digital connectivity she fosters with her family in the Philippines. In fact, this connectivity gave her the boost she needed to continue to work.

Taking into account that "doing family" was not solely a transnational dynamic. Many part-time care workers had some of their family members also live locally in the Bay Area, while others live with fellow care workers they have adopted as fictive kin. The living arrangements with biological and fictive kin found many Filipinos with various jobs and careers in different health professions all under one house. They are employed in a range of health professions, such as nurses, doctors, medical techs, operators, and para-professionals, including CNAs and licensed vocational nurses, and hospital support staff, like janitors. According to Ellen, a care worker who shares a household with her husband and adult daughter and relatives:

> It's a big difference! It's scary in this pandemic, because you don't know if you will get [COVID-19] or not. You know, some people is asymptomatic and you don't know that you're a carrier on that. So I'm afraid for myself. I'm also afraid to the people that I'm taking care of and also, I'm afraid to go to my family. My daughter she is a nurse now. My husband is working as a caregiver at a different place. And we do everything like spraying our shoes. The Clorox wipes, hand sanitizer, putting the mask on, taking off our work clothes right away. That's what the article said; it's hard to breathe with the mask at work. But we're trying our best to support each other. And protect others and protect yourself.

The concerns of care workers about COVID-19 contraction and transmission often revolved around the uncertainty of contracting the virus. However, they demonstrated that their concerns transcend their own ability to work. Rather, they are always hyperaware of contracting and exposing the concentric circles and communities they are a part of. Because of systemic racism and compounding health inequities in communities of color that reduced the accessibility of testing, information dissemination, and protections for Filipino care workers, many of them were navigating the context knowing that it was only a matter of time before they had the virus. In fact, Filipinos on the front lines suffered across the board—one out of three nurses who died from COVID-19 were Filipino. While the tally of how many Filipinos working as health professionals in the United States contracted and died of COVID is inaccessible—due to the lack of data disaggregation for the Asian American community—an educated guess might conclude that tens of thousands of Filipino community members in the United States have died, many of whom were health-care workers on the front lines. While family responsibilities, both transnational and local, shaped how Filipino care workers navigated being on the front lines daily, they demonstrated that their invisibility as essential workers in multiple COVID-19 front lines did not allow them to make decisions that put their health first.

CONCLUSION

The devaluation of care and care work of Filipino caregivers is a logic and practice inherited by a legacy of racialized and gendered history of domestic work in the United States. This legacy translates to a dearth of legal protections for the care workers across racial and ethnic groups. In the United States, this is particularly true when it comes to Filipina/o care workers. Their experiences of fear and uncertainty with regard to their jobs, especially during COVID-19, can be traced to the nation's historical racism toward Black and immigrant working women. In early American history, enslaved Africans and Indigenous people were stolen from their lands and relegated to domestic work in white settler colonists' homes. In and after the US Civil War, Black women could not find jobs outside of domestic work because of employment discrimination and racism in other industries. Domestic work was considered dirty and degrading, with white women often avoiding such jobs, hence racializing the work and the industry for centuries to come. Racist narratives around domestic work informed the stipulations in the 1938 FLSA, which established minimum wage, overtime pay, and other employment standards. In an effort to appease the racist desires of Southern lawmakers to ensure that Black workers could not avail themselves of federal labor protections, domestic workers (and agricultural workers) were purposefully excluded from the FLSA.[18] These historical injustices continue to reverberate into the experiences of care workers now—home care workers are 62 percent people of color, many of whom are Black and immigrant women, and their median income is $16,200.[19] This devaluation of care work has translated to scarce protections and regulations toward an increasingly privatized care industry.

In residential care facilities, those employed may not be formally categorized as "health-care workers" even though they provide vital forms of care labor, such as movement therapy, round-the-clock delivery of medicine, and assistance with daily living activities. Home care workers, such as caregivers to the elderly, personal attendants, and home health aides, are considered essential workers because they provide in-home care for the most vulnerable populations despite lacking sufficient protections for themselves. Although caregivers carry out critical care assistance, residential care facilities have been noted violating various tenets of the FLSA. This has included denying workers' wages and forcing caregivers to work beyond their contracted hours. There is currently no requirement that residential care facilities must have skilled licensed staff onsite or on call, and no legal staffing ratio requirement exists.[20] In California, for example, the Department of Labor and the California Labor Commissioner's Office have found rampant wage and hour violations. Since 2011, caregivers have filed 526 wage theft claims with the Labor Commissioner's Office. Of those cases that went to hearings, workers were found to be owed $2.5 million dollars. However, approximately 71 percent of the judgment amounts due ($1.8 million) remain unpaid.[21]

Furthermore, these limited legal protections extend to home care workers. Domestic workers have been historically excluded by the National Labor Relations Act of 1932. In California, though, standards of the California Occupational Safety and Health Act (Cal/OSHA) require employers to protect their workers from health and safety issues. Workers who provide "household domestic service," which is related to the home care work provided by caregivers, are excluded from these protections.

Limited labor protections greatly affect the health and safety of residential care facility and home care workers. In a study in Boston, Massachusetts, domestic workers faced several health risks. These risks included chronic back pain and exposure to hazardous chemicals, high stress levels on the job, and housing and economic instability.[22] Another study focusing on workers' psychological health in long-term residential care homes revealed how mental health issues were caused by difficult working conditions, disrespect, and discrimination in the workplace.[23] Workers reported health issues from witnessing the suffering and death of their patients and the overload of work due to time pressures and interpersonal demands. Additionally, for immigrant care workers, the lack of labor protections leaves little recourse for workers to file grievances against their employers. Studies have indicated that for migrant care workers, there is a fear of speaking up and being at risk of being fired and deported.[24]

The paradox of Filipino care workers' invisibility under this pandemic does not emerge because of the current conditions; rather, the lack of visibility and protections for Filipino caregivers are a product of ongoing neoliberal and racialized processes in the United States. Highlighting the historical systems of racialized, gendered, and neoliberal patterns that overtly devalue care and care workers in the States helps draw a through line to the current conditions of exploitation for Filipino caregivers. My aim in this chapter is to connect these historical and structural problems to possibly illuminate commonalities among care workers that might lead to solidarity and political organizing.

CHAPTER 3

RELATIONALITY AS A POLITICS OF CARE

Teresa has worked as a caregiver to the elderly in the Bay Area's Silicon Valley for more than a decade. She was an immigrant from the Philippines who left a child and family behind to work in the United States and support her family. Upon her arrival, Teresa became entangled with an employer who coerced her to work alone for twenty-four hours a day as a live-in caregiver with five patients, without anyone to help during the day and through the night shifts. After some months, Teresa knew her work situation could not be right. For some time, she felt hopeless about her situation because her paid work as a caregiver supported her child and many members of her family in the Philippines. If she left her job, she would also be leaving her family without financial support for daily needs. When she demanded to be paid overtime for the hours she was awake to assist her patients, her employer refused and fired her.

Upon meeting organizers from PAWIS in Silicon Valley, Teresa changed her perspective. PAWIS, a Tagalog word that means "sweat" and can be figuratively used to refer to the working class, was an organization that fostered an ethic of care about the well-being of care workers like Teresa. Through PAWIS, Teresa was able to access legal resources to file a wage theft case against her employer with the local Department of Labor—and she won. After her case was settled, Teresa's participation with PAWIS grew. Along with political education sessions, organizing and community-building activities, plenty of time and trips socializing and checking up on caregiver members, she advanced from being just a member to an advanced activist, eventually becoming the vice chairperson of the organization. When I asked Teresa about the importance of political organizing, she answered, "It is important to me because I'm not alone in this, and that I get to take care of *kababayan* [community members] like me." In her record as a worker leader, Teresa has helped with various issues that have come up for workers in PAWIS, from similar cases of wage theft, human trafficking, racial discrimination on the job, cases of abuse and exploitation, and now through difficulties associated with the COVID-19 pandemic. She was literally the poster person of a care worker who has taken her own experiences of tragedy and transformed them into persevering a career in political organizing.

Under the pandemic, the crisis of eldercare was magnified. For caregivers like Teresa and members of PAWIS, the circumstances of the dual crisis of a broken eldercare industry and COVID put many workers at risk with little to no resources to turn to. Elsewhere, Katherine Nasol and I have argued that the pandemic exacerbated the dire conditions in eldercare that led many nursing homes and long-term care facilities to become hot spots for COVID-19 transmission.[1] Teresa reflected on the pandemic's impacts on workers:

> COVID has really increased much, much more of the stress and fears to caregivers. Although even before the pandemic they're already a stress and fears that are already existing but much more in this pandemic. Before, the only fears they have is like losing jobs, or fear of becoming homeless, fears of being deported or raided by the ICE [US Immigration and Customs Enforcement], so all these stresses. But now it's the stress of getting the virus at work or even being a carrier of the virus to their clients. You know, the fear on site is too high, because they don't want to get sick. Caregivers, most of them don't have medical insurance. Employers don't provide medical insurance, and they [caregivers] don't have any.

Teresa described the compounding stressors on caregivers from before and during the pandemic. She mentioned the specter of joblessness, homelessness, and deportation before the global pandemic, and in the next breath,

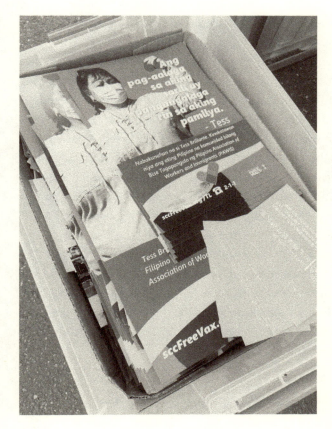

Posters from the Santa Clara County Department of Public Health, 2021, designed to encourage vaccinations in the Filipino Community, in Filipino and English

her comment about the risk for COVID-19 exposure and contraction to their clients demonstrates a concern that is a close second for many caregivers. While caregivers' understanding of the virus early on during lockdown was still inchoate, they were concerned about working with the most vulnerable population: those sixty-five years and older with preexisting conditions. Yet the next set of concerns in Teresa's comments addresses the health of caregivers and their lack of access to health services. Here, her comment is evidence that the dual crisis for care workers that emerged in the pandemic were set in motion from the existing failures in an underfunded and broken industry for long-term care in the United States. This industry knowingly put the health and well-being of caregivers at the bottom of its list of priorities, and therefore, while responding to a global pandemic, caregivers were pushed further down that list.

The lived experiences of Filipino caregivers before the pandemic that were worsened during the pandemic have become the "perfect storm" for those on the front lines of COVID-19. Caregivers remained unseen and invisible frontline workers. The lack of social imagination and structural recognition of care workers, especially in nonhospital settings, deny the many front lines in the time of coronavirus. Given the lack of a federal plan, funds, social infrastructure, and even popular and political narratives about workers in eldercare, caregivers essentially became invisible. The aim of this chapter is to provide evidence that, while caregivers were, and arguably still are, invisible to the American landscape of long-term care, other forms and relationships of perseverance and mutual aid have emerged. The structural failures and absence of reform in the eldercare industry have local and coalitional potential to organize for caregiver rights and welfare. In the following pages, I argue that there are parallel lines in the dual and worsening crisis of caregiving before and during the pandemic along with the types of "communities of care."

COMMUNITIES OF CARE AND PERSISTENCE

Teresa's story anchors us in the ethics and politics of care for the caregivers in this book. I think of Teresa's contributions as a worker leader in creating "communities of care." This term, as I coined and discussed in *The Labor of Care*, refers to the kinds of communities built on the structural location of Filipina domestic workers in New York City in relation to their transnational relationship to their families in the Philippines, the precarity of their domestic employment, and their racialized immigrant experiences in the United States. In this chapter I continue to develop this term and apply it to Filipina care workers in the San Francisco Bay Area. In my research I believe that the theoretical generalizability of "communities of care" is applicable to caregivers in the Bay Area and that this historical moment shapes such experiences in unique ways—namely, through technology and distanced strategies. In fact, I posit that migrant workers like Teresa were already creating the kinds of futures of mutual aid long before the pandemic and, in fact, were able to innovate further under pandemic conditions with the use of technology.

Some aspects of these communities of care are similar. I suggest that the political organizing by Filipino care workers relies on building solidarity rooted in their multiple relationships with care work—from their responsibilities to their biological kin left behind in the Philippines, to the people they care for in their jobs in the United States, to one another in the communities they have with their fellow Filipinas/os in their local communities. In this way, they have activated solidarities on expansive definitions of what Marxist feminists categorize as "social reproductive labor," the type of labor that reproduces society in all aspects with the goal of accumulating capital.[2] Filipino care workers contribute to this reproduction not only by supporting their biological kin but also in their paid work caring for their clients.[3] Moreover, the examples that follow demonstrate that the labor they invest in one another and sustaining their migrant communities unhinges the idea of social reproduction as solely a type of labor that biological kin obliges.[4] Examining the simultaneity of these three dimensions of social reproductive labor untethers such labor from the biological constraints that often hold hostage the popular narrative of "care work." Filipina/o migrants working as caregivers have taken the "perfect storm" of crisis in the industry and in global health as an opportunity to reenvision and reenact social reproductive labor as a nexus of radical care.

At the center of Teresa's story as a migrant mother, care worker, organizer, and Filipina is the entanglement of care and politics. She says, "Caregivers are the most hardworking people, I know. And I always tell people that. Caregiving is not for everybody. If you're not into this, if you don't have the passion to take care of people, you won't last. Not even a month, not even a year. I think of a day of working as a caregiver. Oh, you will give up! So the dedication, you know, to do the work is really unbelievable for a caregiver, especially the Filipino caregivers. They do a lot of sacrifice. It's all because, for the love of the family, you know, that's the motivation of being a caregiver." For her, and many like her, leaving the Philippines is about caring for family members. Working in the domestic work industry is about caring for employers. Activism is about caring for themselves and also their community—their kababayan, as Teresa put it—because of the absence of state supports. This labor in caring for one's self and one's community has often struck me as an unnecessary generosity that care workers extend to one another. After all, they are often concerned about their families in the Philippines and about their own well-being in the United States. Why worry about others in the same boat? And yet, across the precarious domestic work industry, Filipina/o care workers often see their plight intertwined with one another in the United States. Often their ability to support one another is extra, time-intensive labor that they choose beyond the paid and unpaid care work they are already doing.

To understand this dynamic, I apply the term "emotional labor of persistence." Philippine studies scholar Jean Aaron de Borja writes in their recent article about the disruption of life and work for overseas foreign workers under the COVID-19 pandemic.[5] De Borja argues that the frame of "persistence" moves beyond the heroistic narrative of resilience that, in fact, obscures the structural failures that produce Filipino migrant workers' precarity and dispossession. De Borja draws from Filipina American theorist Neferti Tadiar's book *Fantasy Production*, in which Tadiar writes about Filipinos' practice of fate playing in their decisions to migrate and persist elsewhere as *pakikipagsapalaran*.[6] The gamble in migration is an act of faith that many Filipinos try their luck on, hoping for a better future or a different life. In this Filipino word there is an inherent collectivity in one's fate playing. For Filipino migrants who invest in one another, taking on the gamble of working abroad risks experiences of hardship as migrants and workers in precarious positions. Individually, they are betting on themselves as they make their way out in the world, and yet as Tadiar argues, the practice of gambling also comes with *sampalataya*, or "the unarticulated relations among people—feelings, respect, hope and belief."[7] De Borja and Tadiar's theoretical proposition is that these Filipino cultural values and practices govern how Filipino care workers build relationships with one another. The very relations they enact on a daily basis conjure discourses of filial piety, faith, and survival as part and parcel of their collective emotional labor of persistence.

In theorizing the existing and emergent types of collective care in Filipino migrant communities, I acknowledge that persistence can be traced through formal networks such as community organizations and church fellowships. However, I extend the notion of "communities of care" to what Allan Punzalan Isaac, in his book *Filipino Time*, calls the "communality" among Filipino care workers that underscores their interactions and reciprocity.[8] Instead of presuming a unitary and static notion of "community," I center on the reciprocal interactions and practices among care workers. I am able to include the relationships that are not necessarily anticapitalist or explicitly radical or progressive. I recognize the interactions that are temporary and contingent on the historical moment, the immaterial and affective labor of care that is fleeting and ephemeral. In acknowledging the affective dimensions of communality, I cast a wider net to understand the emotional contexts that served as the dense, everyday realities of care workers under COVID-19, experienced individually and, at some level, collectively. With this framing, I link the multitude of care beyond social reproductive labor, or as Isaac puts it, "Operating on the somatic as well as communal level, care work is the creative labor necessary to connect with people, to establish relationship and to project futures for others and ourselves that guide the everyday."[9]

The emergence of radical care and mutual aid in the time of COVID-19 is inextricable from the political economic constraints of neoliberal globalization, racial capitalism, and uncertainty in the time of coronavirus and before. I lift up the emotional labors of persistence and the creative labor of a multitude of care while holding in tension the systematic failures of public health, immigration, and health care in the United States. These broken systems are the preconditions for the communities of care that I highlight in this work. In this chapter, I join scholars who agree that Filipino caregivers endure difficult and arduous work conditions produced by systemic failures in governance and policy.[10] And yet as scholars Hiʻilei Hobart and Tamara Kneese define radical care as a "praxis of radical politics that provides spaces of hope in precarious times,"[11] I consider the concept of "relationality" in the radical care practices among and within Filipino migrant communities as an ethics of caregivers. I ask, What types of radical care are engendered by the systems under which they live and work? What is the affective labor of persistence like when Filipino care workers start creating care strategies for and among one another?

PRECARIOUS POSITIONS AND *KAPWA* EXPLOITATION

Care work as an occupation identifies workers' purpose as chiefly to provide care to their clients; anything besides that relationship to the client is often marked as superfluous, especially because institutions or employers determine care workers' wages solely by the tasks in relation to client care.[12] This transactional definition of labor for caregivers often eclipses many types of care they attend to with regard to their clients, their clients' families, and to one another as coworkers. Because caregiving is defined as a commodity—a transaction for a care worker's labor time in exchange for wages—the devaluation of this work and the potential wage penalty it involves can be attributed to its privatization.[13] Scholars have depicted a range of care work, both paid and unpaid, as reproducing society—in other words, labor for the public good.[14] In various societies, such labor is collectivized and subsidized by state funding, and as the neoliberal state continues to foreclose on social safety nets, work for the public good has become marketized (e.g., costs of rearing children in private or chartered education versus public systems).

Care work is a prime example of the marketization of a public good that results in the precarity and uncertainty of the work. Layered atop global trends of labor migrations, as well as racialized and gendered histories of domestic work in the United States, Filipino care workers are positioned into this industry as low-wage workers, precarious with regard to the domestic industry but also in the nodes of immigration and race.[15] Given the devaluation of care work and care workers, the transactional and marketized nature of caregiving often leaves care workers vulnerable to normalized exploitation in their workplaces, as I discussed in chapter 2. Caregiving is a prime example of how the private and for-profit care industry carry over neoliberal capitalist logics in the work of care. In what follows, I provide examples of how care workers' precarity affects them individually and how it affects their collective acts of faith, perseverance, and persistence.

Caregivers' daily tasks are physically and emotionally draining. The nature of client dependency on one care worker at any given time often creates a process where care workers weigh their clients' emotions over their own in the name of completing their jobs. Miriam, a full-time caregiver, reported how difficult it is working with some clients who are physically aggressive: "We get hurt, you really can't stay away from it. Especially when you have a client who's really active. When he grabs you, [the client] scratches [you]. It's included in the job. You know, when I first walk in here after taking care of the elderly, I thought that you have to be gentle. You have to be slow. You know, when I came here and I stayed in this corner and the whole time I'm like, What did I get myself into?" In her reflections, Miriam's self-alienation distances her from the decisions she has made to come to work as a caregiver. Miriam's expectations did not meet the realities of the physicality of her job, thus inducing self-doubt and anxiety about her ability to do her work. In this "commodification of emotion," Miriam's care work requires her to manage her own internal contradictions, demonstrating what feminist scholars of care have characterized as markers of precarity in paid care work.[16]

Across my research, caregivers have articulated the surprise and shock of just how taxing and challenging it is to assist clients physically and emotionally. Although they recognize that the range of client interactions is a part of their job as caregivers, it often triggers Filipina/o workers to doubt their efficacy. For many, normalizing the physical demands and psychological distress that emerge in the job becomes a way to overcome those doubts. In fact, when caregivers accept pain and physical abuse as "included in the job," as Miriam described, they are accepting that these are occupational hazards compensated with the wage they are given. While they are pushed to the limits in the workplace, Filipina/o care workers persist individually by normalizing the lack of support and training as included in their job description in order to manage psychological distress.[17] They continue their work despite facing extremely difficult situations and emotions.

Filipina/o care workers have indicated that this transactional definition of caregiving is worsened when their employers are also Filipino. I tread carefully here to not lay blame on Filipino exploitation solely on a cultural thesis that Filipinos take advantage of other Filipinos. Rather, I take heed from Filipina American sociologist Jennifer Nazareno's work on the entrepreneurship of Filipina nurses as care home owners and administrators to frame these interactions as a stand-in for a bereft American welfare state.[18] Nazareno argues that Filipino care home owners who are poorly subsidized by the state provide direct care to the vulnerable American aging population and employ care workers. While the insufficient long-term-care funding continues to squeeze these Filipino entrepreneurs, they follow a capitalist logic in relegating care workers to the transactional nature I have discussed above. Often this results in a range of trafficking, exploitation, and abuse by Filipino care home owners at the expense of their Filipino care workers. Although I do not absolve opportunistic Filipino entrepreneurs from exploiting their workers, it is important for me to not rely on a solely cultural explanation for this dynamic. Rather, I aim to contribute a sharper critique of the larger political and economic system that marketizes care work, defunds the long-term care industry, abandons social welfare policies for the chronically sick and elderly, and creates immigration policies that build a disposable labor pool of immigrants to exploit.

To this end, Rica, a full-time, live-in caregiver for a care home with five beds, recounted her first job in the United States:

> Filipino care home owners take a lot of advantage of their kababayan. They really do. Yeah, they should know better. But because they know the worth of a dollar to peso, they know that, like, if they pay you fifty dollars for them it's just fifty dollars, but when you convert to peso, you know, we wouldn't be able—for the life of us, the caregivers wouldn't be able to earn that back home in just an hour. But that's why they can take advantage. They know how much we need the money for family in the Philippines. And so they just keep pressing us.

Rica provides a compelling reason as to why there is rampant exploitation of Filipino care workers by Filipino care home owners. The shared transnational experience and understanding of supporting Philippine-based kin is how care workers explain the co-ethnic exploitation in caregiving. Care workers, some who are recruited from rural provinces in the Philippines, grit their teeth through difficult work conditions because their earnings in dollars go a long way in supporting their families in the Philippines. They are alienated from their labor process because they see their labor time as earnings in pesos. Alongside feelings of obligation, or what many caregivers characterize as *utang ng loob*, the bondage caregivers feel under their co-ethnic employers is a combination of obligation to their families left behind and the opportunity of US employment. This can be a dangerous position for caregivers, as the marketization of caregiving pushes Filipino care home owners to think about their entrepreneurial effort on the basis of profit over the welfare of care workers.

Moreover, Filipino care home owners also rely on Filipino newcomer naivete in their exploitation of Filipino care workers. Alice remembered working for a Filipino couple who recruited three caregivers, including her, directly from their home province in the Philippines:

ALICE: Sometimes there were caregivers who work during the day, and then sometimes they get, they get more time on night shift because they come only at night. That's what happens there, because they wanted to earn some more. But in my case, it happened to me before when I was still working because I live there at the same time. So I don't have the choice but to work there twenty-four hours a day. I didn't even know that it is, it is not right. You know, it's, umm, yeah. Absolutely. I don't even have any day off.

VALERIE: But they pay you for twenty-four hours?

ALICE: Oh, no. They did not. Absolutely, no, they actually, they pay me only—I'll just tell you the figure: six hundred dollars. They only pay me for once a month too. I didn't even know that they were fooling me. I don't even know that. I don't even know how much a caregiver is earning here.

VALERIE: So sorry. Yeah, that is very low. And you stayed there for six months and you had no idea?

ALICE: Yes, because I didn't know anything about America, about fairness in caregiving. I stayed there for one year and one month.

Alice was nearly fifty-two years old when she was recruited from the Philippines. Her daughters were entering high school, so she felt the need to work abroad to fund their collegiate goals. A housewife and occasional domestic worker in her province, Alice came to the United States with an expectation to work but without a network of people to inform her of standard work policies, wages, and worker rights. For Alice and her fellow recruits, free lodging and food and a monthly paycheck were what they signed up for and what they received. Their travel documents were withheld and access to other caregivers who could compare notes in terms of wages and work conditions were limited, thus making their Filipino employers the only trustworthy sources of information. This kind of isolation creates an environment of precarity and vulnerability that can, in fact, be interpreted as "human trafficking."

The experiences of a number of care workers in this study fit into a broad definition of human trafficking in that they were recruited with the promise of good salaries but had been relegated to "force, fraud, and coercion" upon arrival in the United States.[19] In the case of Filipino migrant workers, trafficking is complicated by the debt bondage that they enter into with recruitment agencies or individual recruiters when they leave the Philippines.[20] The care workers in this study who came through various avenues of recruitment and temporary visas have similar experiences. Rina, a forty-year-old caregiver, recounted her experience:

> I am a caregiver here in the Bay Area. I came here in December of 2007. I worked as a hotel housekeeper and front desk because we were hired from the Philippines as hotel workers and my contract was a year. So I was assigned in Florida but the entrance was kinda illegal because they processed everything. We have a notice to start work and there was an approval from [the Department of] Labor. I entered as a H-2B [temporary nonagricultural] unskilled worker, so my contract is one year. Before my one-year contract expired at the hotel, I moved to California because my company said that there is work here. I had a friend from the company, a caregiver in Danville, said they had a vacancy. So I left the company and my friend said, "Do you like to be sponsored by the Filipino care home owner? Come to this job." So I moved. But after I filed for a sponsorship with the Filipino owner and the lawyer, the lawyer said that there's a fee and it's not free. And my employer would take the money from my check monthly. And the case is ongoing because they don't know if the visa from my employer will come through, there

is no assurance. So I have to stay with my employer for the visa and to pay for the lawyer.

Rina's story of being trafficked to work in the US hotel industry and ending up in the caregiving industry is common in my study. Trafficking cases of Filipino workers imported from the Philippines as nurses or steel workers have been on the rise in the past decade and a half.[21] The care workers in my research in the past decade have turned to caregiving as a de facto occupation as their legal cases are being processed or as undocumented people whose temporary guest-worker visas have expired.

Migrant workers rely on immigrant social networks to secure work as caregivers, like Rina did. However, they become stuck in a legal limbo in terms of legal status at entry and then undocumented status upon understanding the coercive nature of their contracts. But even worse, as working migrants, they are not recognized as trafficked persons, given their entrance with visas and their ability to find and continue to work "illegally" in the United States. Annie Fukushima proposes that this labor migration of Asian workers fits a historical pattern of importing cheap racialized labor that obscures present-day US schemes of human labor trafficking.[22] While the only legible subjects that can be treated as "trafficked" are those who fit the model of being brought to work in the United States under the guise of "force, fraud, and coercion," Filipino care workers who have made constrained decisions to leave their original recruitment agencies to work as caregivers cannot often be recognized by the state as legitimately vulnerable, and therefore they urgently need assistance.[23] Many Filipino care workers like Rina, Alice, and even Teresa (from the beginning of this chapter) were technically trafficked by Filipino recruiters and care home owners, but because of their co-ethnic reliance on one another, these cases do not get picked up as "trafficking cases" and thus run rampant in the caregiving industry.

The Filipino cultural value of *kapwa* can be characterized as a worldview wherein a Filipina/o sees oneself as inextricable from the "generalized other." Reflecting the collectivistic nature of Filipino culture, in opposition to individualistic tendencies in Western cultures, kapwa is an outlook that undergirds Filipinos' belief in a social belonging and a relatedness to one another in terms of interactions and relationships.[24] And yet the examples

I have shown demonstrate that kapwa can be used to create hierarchical power relations between Filipinos toward the end of accumulating profit over the welfare of their fellow Filipinos. While the outlook of kapwa and other cultural values like utang ng loob (an obligation and social reciprocity) and *tiis* (grit and determination) can compound to produce precarious positions for Filipino caregivers and wielded as values of domination by Filipino care home owners and entrepreneurs, it is important to understand that these cultural tropes are not ahistorical. They do not exist in a vacuum. In fact, they are deployed as strategies in the caregiving industry, much like other transnational industries that include recruitment of Filipinos in the Philippines and delivery of low-wage workers to high-demand markets all over the world as the mechanics of a labor export regime that has lasted and evolved many times since the 1970s. Further back than the neoliberalization of migration in the Philippines, Filipino American psychologists suggest that the damage to ideals of kapwa can be traced to Spanish colonialism, wherein Filipinos internalized the idea that feudal and hierarchical structures between co-ethnics are conditioned by class and social status.[25]

And still the damage to kapwa has a different iteration as Filipino Americans and Filipino migrants faced virulent racism as they worked and made their lives in the United States.[26] The American racial order, one that pits Filipinos against one another, has been a process of learning that class is a marker of dignity enshrined by race. This global racial ideology is one that traveled to the Philippines with US military occupation, neocolonization, and imperial dominance. As Filipino migrants, entrepreneurs, and care workers recreate hierarchies of power in the United States, they have internalized one another's differential value in relation to the "American Dream," which likely allows for exploitation if profit and success in the States is the goal. Kapwa exploitation works from what Katherine Nasol calls a "neoliberal governance of care" that protects American racial capitalism and the hierarchies of value that are assigned to Filipino, immigrant, people of color whose low-wage work bolsters the subsistence of aspirational middle-class Filipinos.[27] While what the eye can see realizes that Filipinos are exploiting other Filipinos, I join feminist Filipinx scholars in insisting that these co-ethnic interactions be contextualized in the political economy of care under racial capitalism.

RELATIONAL CARE AND PAKIKIPAGSAPALARAN

In a stifling industry of caregiving, Filipina migrants are often defined and valued for their caring for their clients. Central to this construction of the Filipina as the "best" caregiver is a long-standing racial and gendered construction of Asian Americans for different labor markets in the United States.[28] The particularity of a caregiver's job—for example, the kinds of assistance they provide or the therapies they assist with—determines their retention in their position. In fact, caregivers' ability to attend to the very particular and repetitive tasks of their jobs often leads to exploitation and abuse, because the range of care practices they actually do are rarely recognized and compensated. Instead of defining their work and their value based on the particularities of their jobs, I invoke the idea of "relational care" from Joan Tronto's work in reconsidering the flaws in "caring institutions" to consider how radical strategies of care have emerged from caregivers' practices in their workplaces and in their communities. The story that follows illustrates some of the advantages in considering care workers' lives in terms of relational care.

Carmela, Nanet, and Sylvia shared a one-bedroom apartment that they occupied at different times during a work week. Sometimes there would be one person in the apartment for two or three days at a time, and at times two of them would overlap as they came and went to their partial live-in caregiving jobs in Silicon Valley. It was special when all three women were together in their apartment. On those days, the trio of middle-age Filipinas would cook their favorite Filipino dishes, sing karaoke, and talk about the children and grandchildren they had left behind in the Philippines. They became friends when they met up at a nearby Catholic church, and their living arrangement had worked out for several years now.

During the onset of the pandemic, all three of them tried to keep each other updated through text messages regarding the new, and sometimes frightening, conditions of their work. They often scoured the websites of city agencies and then called one another when they found resources for PPE such as masks and nitrile gloves or food banks. Early on in the pandemic, Carmela and Nanet were worried about Sylvia, since they hadn't received a text message from her one day, which was quite unusual. All three of them had overlapped at their shared apartment just two days before, making sure that they all had PPE for when they went into work. Carmela and Nanet decided they would start calling Sylvia's coworkers, splitting up the contacts they knew of between the two of them. The first round of coworkers hadn't had a shift for a few days, and on their second round of calls to the Filipino caregivers at Sylvia's facility, they learned that she had been sent to a hotel to quarantine because she tested positive for COVID-19. But Sylvia's coworker who informed them of the situation did not know the name of the hotel.

Worried, Carmela and Nanet started to call the hotels near Sylvia's workplace, and finally they found a hotel with her name listed in one of the rooms. As soon as they were patched into her room, they asked why she wasn't responding on her phone. Sylvia quickly explained that she did not have her phone charger when she was committed to the hotel by the facility owner in order to quarantine. She expressed her fears about the virus to Carmela and Nanet. She had lost her sense of taste and smell and felt feverish and tired, but beyond that she was okay. The three women chatted about the anxiety of not being able to earn a wage, for how long? Would Sylvia be terminated? What would happen to her family in the Philippines? COVID was not first on Sylvia's priority list—she knew she would survive it. But losing her job? Her family might not survive that.

Sylvia kept apologizing to her housemates and friends for not trying to get in touch with them sooner, and that is when Carmela and Nanet started to realize that they, too, might have been exposed to the virus when they were all at their apartment just a few days earlier. Sylvia insisted that they get their COVID tests and call in sick from work right away. Both Carmela and Nanet did just that, while shortly thereafter they dropped off some Filipino baked goods and Sylvia's phone charger at her door. Wracked with nerves and anxiety, Nanet and Carmela decided they would quarantine at their apartment, away from their clients at work and friends, as they awaited their test results. Similar to the package they delivered to Sylvia, Carmela and Nanet found a package of Filipino food and baked goods at their apartment door, organized by Sylvia through their church fellowship. Fortunately, a few days later, Carmela and Nanet tested negative for COVID-19. After an additional seven days of quarantine, they were able to go back to work.

In this story of Filipino care workers in the throes of the pandemic, two points are illustrated: first, women-centered, immigrant support networks have existed for Filipina migrants working as home care workers. These "communities of care" have operated on the common experiences of Filipinas as migrant mothers, low-wage care workers, and racialized immigrants in the United States.[29] Carmela, Nanet, and Sylvia's shared apartment is not an uncommon domicile for home care workers who maintain different types of live-in, full-time, or part-time jobs as caregivers to the elderly. The cost of sharing a living space allows migrant home care workers to save on their monthly bottom line, which is often the difference between their US living costs and remittances for their families in the Philippines. Outside of communal living arrangements, many church fellowships, regional organizations, and workers' rights organizations have operated to assist migrant home care workers with practical matters from immigration assistance to medical help. These communities of care are punctuated by home care workers' shared identities wherein solidarities can often be mobilized toward activism and leadership.[30] In what Neferti Tadiar discusses as pakikipagsapalaran, she argues that when faced with similar compounding conditions, this cultural value and Filipino word captures the fighting approach Filipinos take on to face what can seem like insurmountable challenges.[31] I argue that the care Filipina migrants carve out for one another is pakikipagsapalaran—a way to acknowledge the compounding weights and external conditions of power that constrain their lives and, notably, the multiple ways they can provide care and receive care from one another.

Second, under a global health crisis, and working within a poorly funded US eldercare industry, many migrant care workers fell victim to the lack of infrastructure to inform and protect the invisible frontliners at the vanguard of assisted living facilities for the elderly. As noted earlier, those most vulnerable to COVID-19 are people sixty-five or older with preexisting conditions.[32] Still, it was the communities of care who scaffolded the lives of Filipino migrant home care workers and aided them during their times of need. As Carmela and Nanet looked for Sylvia to provide her with immediate needs like a phone charger and comfort food, they remind us that many migrant women of color doing the work of caregiving are here on their own, with much of their biological family in the Philippines. Thus, the care and mutual aid that becomes activated depends on a reconceptualization of care into one that accepts relationality to foster different strategies of pakikipagsapalaran.

PERSISTENCE THROUGH PRECARITY

The bonds that caregivers build with one another embody the "emotional labor of persistence," a concept that Philippine studies scholar Jean de Borja discusses in terms of Filipino migrant workers under COVID-19.[33] In their study, de Borja relies on the idea of pakikipagsapalaran to explain that the collective will of caregivers draws from their future-oriented outlook for themselves, their families, and one another. Still, what does it look like in their daily lives? The mutual care Filipina migrants provide to each other through both material and emotional means is enveloped in an intimate understanding of the stakes in their jobs. Miriam, a full-time caregiver, told a story about the pain of loss that is an understated part of the caregiving profession and how she shares that pain with other caregivers:

> Emotionally you're gonna get attached to your client and time comes that they have to go. They get sick. The very first time I had my client and she passed, that really hit me hard. That was really hard and there's three of us working with her and we're all high school friends, so we all cry because she was a very sweet lady. Very sweet lady, so we all, you know, cried with each other. And it's like I said, I don't feel like taking care of again, but now it's where your heart is and I keep going back every time. And I took care of a few more, and they all die.

Care workers for the elderly realize that employers with whom they build relationships will undoubtedly pass away. Therefore, Miriam's pain of losing a client whom she deeply cared for is one that can only be shared with her coworkers who can relate to the strange conditions of working for someone, building a close emotional bond, and then accepting that they are shepherding clients to their final states.

Miriam's comment displays the importance of her friends and co-caregivers to cope with such grief. She described her reticence about taking care of older clients in the future because of the sadness she had felt in the past and because she knew she would feel it again. However, Miriam has continued to work as a caregiver with the inevitability of her future clients' deaths. One prevailing reason she has continued is because of the community that helps her care for herself in times of grief. The trio of caregivers who cried together, said a final farewell to their client together, and urged one another to continue in care work is a persistence I have seen over and over again in the lives and experiences of caregivers. While such resilience may be an avenue for co-regulation and interpersonal coping strategies in the moment, these support systems can also lead to a greater ability in self-regulation and individual coping in the future.

Another example of how caregivers understand and enact the emotional labor of persistence with and for one another, especially during the pandemic, can be demonstrated by Richelle, a part-time caregiver who holds multiple jobs in the Bay Area. After being asked, "Why do you caregivers help other caregivers out?" Richelle responded:

> Because we share the same experiences. But the thing is, I, I know it's some things are easier said than done. So it's a given. Filipinos have compassion, a little bit more compassion to their fellow Filipino. When you're a caregiver, you have to use your compassion, your tiis, *lalo na*, especially under COVID. We know that we are in danger, we know, we know our family is depending on us, though. So we pass along the info we have. You give extra shields and masks if you have.

Indeed, having a shared experience of being a caregiver and a Filipino migrant is "easier said than done," as Richelle struggled to articulate the commonality among her peers. Yet the persistence in finding that commonality in an effort to be of assistance to one another was something Richelle was so sure of—in her words, "it's a given." This insistence on compassion and kindness, regardless of the precarious conditions of their own work or immigration status, has been prominent in my research over the last fifteen years for Filipino nannies, housekeepers, caregivers, and personal attendants. Perhaps my astonishment at this generosity comes from knowing the various exploitation and abuse many Filipino migrants endure in their work, and yet they are the first in line to stand up for one another. Their persistence to kapwang Pilipino—to recognize and actualize the blurring of self and other, even under the most difficult of conditions—exemplifies pakikipagsapalaran.

Markedly, the pandemic, and all of the uncertainty it presented for caregivers, as Richelle demonstrated in her quote, increased the need for material and emotional support across the ranks of Filipino care workers. This community of care was directly responding to the increased danger of contraction and transmission of the COVID-19 virus. In Richelle's comment, she intertwines the idea of risk in her job with the larger fate of her family in the Philippines. Filipino migrant workers' collective imagination around families in the Philippines becomes the driving motivation for the pakikipagsapalaran—a joint effort in ensuring that fellow care workers have the shields and masks necessary to continue on in their jobs, because, after all, many had families in the Philippines to support. This support across workplaces is crucial, especially when many friends and family in the Philippines are suffering from COVID restrictions and the loss of work.

When asked how caregivers found the time and initiative to help one another, Julia, a full-time caregiver in an assisted facility, explained:

> Kasi nga, no man's island, kailangan talaga, kailangan mag tulong sa isat-isa. Para lalong gumaan ang trabaho, kasi mahirap yung lost ka diba? Pag punta mo sa isang place like this, di alam yung consequences nung isang desisyon mo. And mga ibang Ate na caregiver, syempre, the same thing din, mga TNT dati, nawalan ng trabaho, walang alam so COVID COVID, ano yon? Di talagang sigurado kung ano sinasabi nila so at least sa isa't isa kakagaan ng loob na tulungan lang. Kahit konting advice. Nakakalighten, nakaka tulong.
>
> Because no man's an island, it's really needed, you need to help out one another. So that the work will get lighter, because it's so hard when you're lost, right? When you come to a place like this, you don't know all the consequences of your decision. And other *Ates* other Filipinas with more experience as a caregiver. Of course, the same thing, they were undocumented, they got laid off in the past, they don't know anything

about COVID. What is that? They're not sure what is the right info given to us, so at least with one another we can ease one another's worry by helping. Even a little advice, you can feel more at ease, you can help others too.

Here, we can see the caring relationships that sustain Julia. Chief among those are other Filipina caregivers—referring to them as "Ates," a word of respect for older women—who have become a source of mutual abundance for one another, providing them with the space to receive and give support to one another, their emotional labor of persistence is caught up in their relationships with one another. Especially when their typical social support systems are far away and when global stressors like COVID-19 require constant sounding boards for new adjustments at work.

In Julia's comment, I find that her references to other caregivers' pasts as unemployed or undocumented becomes one way that many can relate to one another, and although the advice and support does not often translate to legal pathways, the emotional labor of persistence based on one's past is a powerful way of caring for one another. There is no English translation accurate enough to capture *nakakagaan ng loob*; the literal translation would be that another person helps to lift the weight in one's spirit. In my interpretation, I've translated the word to "ease," which does not do justice for the gravity of this exchange and this clause. But here, in this collective lifting of burdens, is the emotional labor of persistence, where past experiences of hardship give way to future possibilities of care for one another.

RELATIONAL CARE IN ACTIVISM

Teresa, a worker leader for PAWIS in Silicon Valley whose comments open this chapter, connects her own experience of exploitation as a caregiver when she worked at a four-bed facility for twenty-four hours a day for months on end. She found a Filipino migrant organization that assisted her in assessing her work conditions and, finally, in mounting a wage theft case for the work she had not been compensated for. Later, Teresa became a leader in the organization using her own experience as a platform to organize and mobilize other caregivers:

> The activism is very important to me because it can lead to—it can lead the workers to really seek for a change. For example, like me, talking through my experience—if I didn't join the community, PAWIS, I won't be able to know my rights as a worker. So when I learned all my rights, then that pushed me to, okay, seek justice for myself. It's not just enough to learn, or to know your rights; it's more of the guts to really fight. And that's something you don't learn in school or, you know, it's through experience. I have the experience and then I have the people! I share experience with people, I see that I'm not alone in this kind of situation, and, you know, I saw them. Some work and they step up and fight for their rights, so it's the same in the community. You do what people has done, like caregivers, the new ones, maybe they'll learn from us as well.

Here, I highlight Teresa's comment about the basis for her activism in a grassroots migrant worker organization for Filipinos in the Bay Area because she speaks of this strategy as a form of collective well-being. Scholars have proposed that Teresa's experiences are rooted in a "politics of care" that "draw[s] on rich interdisciplinary traditions and social movements to theorize and practice care as an inherently interdependent survival strategy, a foundation for political organizing, and a prefigurative politics for building a world in which all people can live and thrive."[34] Teresa starts from her own experience, remembers the political education she received, the agitation she felt from her consciousness-raising process. Then she acknowledges her ability to link her experience to others, all of which is undergirded by an ethic of care for new and future caregivers in her community. Her politics of care goes beyond an interpersonal relationship with other caregivers, spilling over to her ability to connect survival strategies to an impetus for continuous political organizing.

I have shared evidence that horizontal care fostered among caregivers in their workplace is often in response to the unequal power relations in the paradoxically uncaring institutions they work for.[35] Issues in the workplace such as wage theft, unsafe working conditions, and exploitation result in caregivers feeling shame, thus isolating themselves from one another. When their fellow caregivers do not know what to do when workplace abuse arises, or when care workers distance themselves from a coworker who has attracted undue attention to themselves, the social bonds between Filipina/o migrants thin out. Some might not want to implicate themselves due to fear of retaliation or just plain fear. Filipino caregivers who experience loneliness and isolation at their workplaces depend on community gathering spaces to find respite. Church and fellowship, Filipino restaurants and shopping centers, community centers and Filipino ethnic events all served as social gathering places, a relief from the isolation of caregiving work. Caregivers used these spaces to exchange information about jobs, housing, and current events. There, they would celebrate their milestones and birthdays and remit money to their families in the Philippines. This social support network was a robust one that served pragmatic and leisurely purposes. All of this happened before the pandemic.

During the COVID-19 pandemic, though, the characteristic of isolation for caregivers was exacerbated. Before the pandemic, some caregivers might have integrated into their weekly routines movies or meet-ups with other caregivers and patients for a walk at a park or a nearby mall. With the lockdowns, however, caregivers and their patients were unable to leave their premises. Given the population they serve, public places became dangerous for their patients. While their work routines stayed the same, intensifying as news of the virus spread, their communal spaces and events disappeared. This lack of contact among community members foreclosed the opportunity to exchange information about the pandemic. Basic information regarding the virus and how to protect oneself was placed on the shoulders of individual caregivers. What caregivers could expect from their employers in terms of safety and health protections was limited to what employers communicated to their employees. The opportunity to learn what other caregivers were demanding from their employers, and perhaps what employers were willing to provide, was further limited because of caregivers' lack of communal spaces.

As the world turned to Zoom and videoconferencing to transition to remote work and school, caregivers were at a loss. They were not considered a workforce that could opt out of coming into their workplaces. They were essential workers, as they provided critical care for their clients. The hours Filipina/o migrants worked in care homes intensified because caregivers felt the charge of protecting their patients from COVID-19. Yet if there were

Zoom training for caregivers to prepare them for the nuances and changes in the pandemic, they did not have quick access to computers, or training to learn virtual platforms. Additionally, many Filipino caregivers, who are generally between forty-five and fifty-five years old, did not always have the same technological literacy and dexterity as younger generations, who might better adapt to pandemic technologies.

Still, it was the innovation of PAWIS to address these issues that became a powerful pivot in our research and community organizing collaboration. Early in the pandemic, one way to keep in touch with caregivers in the PAWIS organization was through group text apps like GroupMe or WhatsApp. But soon enough, PAWIS worker leaders were convinced that the lockdown and the pandemic would last for more than just a short period, and therefore the organization explored how to convene their members through Zoom. PAWIS leaders activated a Filipino cultural practice called, *kapihan*, or a coffee break, loosely translated into English as monthly Zoom events for caregivers.

Although the virtual Zoom space was not the same as in-person socializing, caregivers, and many Filipino immigrants before them, were already familiar with translating some of their day-to-day lives into some digital and virtual format, given their relationships with their families in the Philippines are mediated by ICTs like Facebook, FaceTime, and Instagram. The kapihan events not only sought to create social spaces for caregivers to connect; they also offered practical advice from labor lawyers with regard to navigating fast-changing federal and state-level benefits for unemployment or paycheck assistance. Both the opportunity to connect with other caregivers and access to legal advice were compelling reasons to get together. Even though Zoom required Filipino caregivers to learn a new app and troubleshoot connectivity in their workplaces, PAWIS worker leaders committed to train their members by phone.

In this example, I argue that political organizations like PAWIS, which focuses on advocating for Filipino workers and immigrant rights in Silicon Valley, become beacons of light for caregivers who are experiencing exploitation and abuse. But they also provide care and social support that is crucial to caregivers for their information and support regarding issues in the workplace. Athena is a caregiver who has been a member of PAWIS and an advocate of extending the organization's resources to Filipino migrants who might need their assistance: "For me," she says, "show the caregivers [PAWIS] so that they will become aware of what is happening. They will also feel that they are not the only ones who are facing these kinds of problems so that they will not be afraid to approach organizations like PAWIS that help them out. They will know that there are really other caregivers who get abused." In this comment, Athena is invoking a sense of intelligibility among caregivers who might have similar experiences of exploitation and abuse. That sense of shared experience can be a possible source of strength and solidarity. As we think through the plurality of care in the lives of low-wage workers, who are often pressured for every moment of care work they can provide to their clients, we find that these very same care workers possess a well of empathy and compassion toward one another. The intelligibility offered by Athena is not only a way to recognize the humanity in another but also a possibility in building a bridge to care for many unknown Filipina/o migrants working as caregivers in the present and the future.

In another instance, a Filipina caregiver, Rina, who was actively involved with Filipinos Advocating for Justice (FAJ) in the East Bay Area, commented on the role of organizations in providing social support to migrants. Rina had been active with FAJ before the pandemic and continued to stay involved during the lockdown period of the pandemic. Rina said:

RINA: The advantage with being with FAJ, is that we see and talk to each other virtually. Recently, we were talking to each other, asking how each other is doing right now.
INTERVIEWER: Would you say your main community is from FAJ? Or from church?
RINA: I have community from FAJ of caregivers that I met when I was working in Danville. I also have an active support from my church friend because before I don't work weekends and I can go to church. But on Saturdays we have an activity where we go door knocking *dito sa* here in the Bay Area. We do this and after, of course, we become friends. You know, before COVID we used to just hang out together. We

go to Jollibee or Seafood City because one of our friends had a car and she would take us and then drop us at the bus stop after our day off. So things like that, we enjoy ourselves.

The politics of care that is built through relationships and trust here is phenomenal. And it is important to note that the practice of communality also centers on joy and lightheartedness. On days off or time off, when many other workers could be maximizing their time to earn wages in part-time positions, Rina shows that a part of why she has become a part of these political organizations is that she, and her comrades, enjoy one another.

The practice of joy cannot be understated as an essential facet of communities of care. Organizations like PAWIS and FAJ provide multiple outlets of care and different receptivities of care. From waging campaigns for rights or providing a space where care workers can connect with one another and enjoy each other's company, the multiple directions of care are boundless. It is significant to note that it is care workers in this study who have repeatedly characterized these forms of social support and political organizing methods as forms of care. Their descriptions of kapwa and belonging mark these relationships as robust with communality—interactions that build trust, care, and hope. Similarly, in her book *Care Activism*, Ethel Tungohan argues that these types of "subversive friendships" among Filipino migrant care workers in Canada affirm workers' need and commitment to building relationships with one another.

Creating multiple communities of care from within their workplaces and community organizations is crucial in helping to fulfill the needs of Filipino workers. Ian, a caregiver who is not a member of a formal Filipino migrant worker organization, said:

> In the Filipino community, maybe there's a way they can update the system to reach out to our kababayans here. More than what they are doing right now. And hopefully they can create more organizations, Filipino organizations that help Filipinos who are still struggling with unemployment and especially with housing. . . . And hopefully they can create an association that will provide the needs of Filipinos, especially medical—

they can create a clinic for mainly Filipinos. That's it. With the situation now, everyone's separated, not knowing where to go.

Ian described the need to support Filipinos who are struggling with unemployment, lack of housing, and medical support, especially during the COVID-19 pandemic. He pointed out that an organization outside of his workplace, outside of government programs, might be able to provide the level of support many caregivers need. I argue that the multiple experiences of caregivers—some who are already members of community organizations and those who aren't—show that many caregivers do not see governmental institutions or even their employers and workplaces as resources for support. Rather, they have identified that for those who are often made invisible, care can and does exist in their own communities and political organizations—and that perhaps when care is seen beyond the transactional nature, compounded by structurally broken care industries, the plurality of care among workers and their communities can offer a radical vision about caring for one another.[36]

Scholars have taken the concept "community of care," from my first book, *The Labor of Care*, to demonstrate how Filipino migrant workers—from diasporic locations such as Canada, the United Kingdom, Italy, and Hong Kong—have enacted and innovated care work among each other and especially under the COVID-19 pandemic.[37] Across the globe, studies describe how the conditions of precarity and exploitation were worsened during the pandemic because of Filipino migrants' lack of access to health care, legalization, and political inequalities germane to the country where they live. Also, in agreement with what I found in my research, Filipino migrants in the diaspora have turned to advocacy and community organizations for both assistance and, more important, an ongoing ethic of care that is aimed at identifying and circulating the needed resources of domestic workers among themselves. While providing services and establishing nonprofit organizations can lend themselves to capitulation into a neoliberal governance, I argue that there is potential for these horizontal practices of care—the building of communities of care—to have a radical resonance that can be critical of systems of power.

CONCLUSION

In my work, both political and academic, the questions that guide my inquiry in the intersection of "care" and "politics" begin with what Shellee Colen has called "stratified reproduction"—a concept that has helped me understand that the ongoing commodification of care work amplifies already existing stratification based on race, ethnicity, class, gender, and sexuality on a global scale.[38] This concept has led me to always start in the place where care workers in the United States, a majority of whom are ethnic immigrant women of color, come from: the Global South. Filipinas have become the prime subject for a global commodification of care workers. For the care workers in my study, before they even make it to the Philippine international airport in Manila, Filipinas are already conceptualized and targeted as potential low-wage care workers for domestic markets in the United States, Canada, Europe, the Middle East, and across the Asia-Pacific region. The systemic nature of neoliberal sending states exporting their citizens is not a new idea, but it has been solidified as a characteristic of contemporary globalization.[39]

As I mature into roles as a researcher, scholar, activist, and mother, who has continued to do systematic research in the communities of Filipina/o domestic workers, it behooves me to complicate my sociological analysis with the textures, temporalities, and intimacies that emerge in my participant observations and kuwentuhan. In his work on time and affective labor, Filipino cultural studies theorist Allan Punzalan Isaac argues, "The inherent creativity that is part of contemporary care labor generates unquantifiable vital forms in everyday work and living."[40] In fact, care workers in my study before and after the COVID-19 lockdown, and throughout the pandemic's restrictions, innovated practices of caring for one another that were not allowed by their employers, were abandoned by American governmental agencies, or were disregarded by Philippine consular offices. Even prior to the pandemic, care workers pooled together money in lending circles for the times when natural disasters like typhoons and earthquakes hit their hometowns.

During the pandemic, they learned how to operate new technologies like Zoom so that they could stay in touch about lifesaving information and to check in about how everyone was doing. As restrictions lifted, they organized a pragmatic form of assistance—to distribute PPE widely to their fellow care workers—*and* they baked banana bread to go into the care packages they dropped off at the porches of care homes that employ Filipina caregivers. Isaac writes, "Care work is creative labor necessary to connect with people, to establish relationships, and to project futures for others and ourselves."[41] The point is that we cannot just see care workers at the intersection of exploitation and abuse, as laboring bodies in the global and transnational production of domestic work. They are as much in the throes of those systemic problems as they are creators of new political subjectivities, fostering a multitude of human capacities to distribute and receive the care that is incommensurate with how value is defined in late-stage capitalism. And in this work, in their ethics of care, I think of Tita Teresa's contributions as a worker leader in creating "communities of care" and how migrant workers like her are already creating the kinds of futures we are dreaming up in political social movements and intellectual discourses.

Building on my past conceptualization of "communities of care," Filipina care workers take from their multiple relationships with care work: from their responsibilities to their kin left behind in the Philippines, to the people they care for in their jobs in the United States, to one another in their organizing communities. In this multidirectionality of care they have realized expansive definitions of care work, and they have used these opportunities to reenvision their labor as a nexus of radical care.

CHAPTER 4

KUWENTUHAN AND INTERGENERATIONAL ACTIVISM

As I peered into the Filipino Community Center on Mission Street in San Francisco one crisp fall evening in 2012, lights and laughter in the main hall welcomed me into one of our kuwentuhan sessions. At least forty people were busy hugging and catching up, shuffling papers into neat packets, arranging chairs into threes, and setting up the food table filled with Filipino dinner dishes in time for our meeting at 6:00 p.m. As I walked in with my folder in hand, ready to facilitate the kuwentuhan—or talk-story—sessions, I was greeted with warmth in boisterous calls of "*Kamusta*?" and jokes like "Almost late to class, *Profesora!*"

Before I could put my bag down, two Filipino American youth, Ronald and Abigail (both pseudonyms), approached me to check in about the technology and volunteer logistics of the session. They reassured me that all the recording devices were set up, tested, and ready to record the conversations we had planned to have that evening. We were short one recording device, but Ronald was ready to sit with one trio and set up his computer with a microphone to record their kuwentuhan session and troubleshoot any tech issues. Big exhale. I was relieved that he had already come up with a solution for the unexpected problem. Abigail reminded the volunteers to check in and told them that after dinner we would have a short briefing about the roles of volunteers during kuwentuhan. The volunteers were Filipina American women in their twenties to thirties who were leaders and members in a progressive women's organization called GABRIELA San Francisco and Filipino American students with the League of Filipino Students at San Francisco State University (SF State) and Kasamahan at the University of San Francisco. As I looked around, I saw that the young people were already sitting with their dinner plates and talking with the care workers in attendance. Laughter and chatter filled the air.

Without a doubt, the CARE Project kuwentuhan sessions focused on the lives and experiences of Filipino care workers. As one of the scholar-activists working collaboratively with the center's workers' rights program and the care worker themselves, I found the logistics and details to be quite overwhelming, at times falling between my fingers. So, the time and labor of young people who volunteered their evenings and weekends to the project's purpose was invaluable. Many Filipina American professionals and graduate students who were GABRIELA members sought to take part in the research project because so many care workers were Filipina immigrants, and Filipina/o students were excited to participate in the project because they were keen on learning from and building solidarity with migrant workers. Their intrinsic motivation to offer their time and knowledge stemmed from their parallel political conscientization and willingness to invest in migrant worker power in our local community. Just as Filipina/o care workers volunteered their time and labor to the project for the same purpose, the reciprocal community building effort lifted the spirit of *bayanihan*, a spirit of collective effort in our program. When the kuwentuhan session started, two care workers would follow a kuwentuhan guide with the very themes we had decided on during our previous research trainings. Volunteers would take notes and help to manage the recording technology during the conversation, scheduled to last thirty to forty minutes. As we began the session, the young people in the room adjusted volumes on devices, clarified terminology from the themes in the guide, interpreted from Tagalog to English and back again, and laughed and cried as the stories were told.

The CARE Project at the Filipino Community Center was one of the most transformative experiences I have had as a scholar and activist. Crafting a research process with Filipina/o community organizers, worker leaders, youth, students, and professionals, a majority of them women and queer, was exhilarating and exhausting. I was excited to step away from the isolation of academia and ensure that many different stakeholders were involved in creating a project that would benefit the care workers in our community. The project felt like we were organizing a large-scale, sustained, community-building event; rather, it was a process that took over a year to accomplish. As one of the scholar-activists who had experience with a community-engaged research project such as this, I felt the need to try to make sure that all groups involved had a democratic voice in the process. There was also the logistics of the meetings, outreach to care workers, food and drink, pickup and drop-off for disabled and elderly care workers, recording sessions, transcription and storage, developing research methods materials that were appropriate for community members who were full-time workers, charting out the research program and recalibrating timelines. It required a bayanihan effort—an effort that required an entire community to pursue and achieve a goal.

I was encouraged by not only care workers committed to the weekly meetings and preparation work for the kuwentuhan sessions but also how they showed up to the workshops, all of which happened after work hours. And yet I felt nervous that centering on the lives and work of care workers in the Filipino community in San Francisco would dampen the interest of college students and working professionals who had volunteered in the early stages of the CARE Project. In fact, it was their dedication that also humbled me. Care workers clearly saw a benefit in sharing their experiences in kuwentuhan. A sense of collectivity emerged when one care worker shared a story and another care worker resonated with that experience of abuse and exploitation or survival and victory. The CARE Project also explicitly developed leadership among the care worker ranks via parallel political education sessions, so the care workers could increase their capacity to deepen their leadership skills and knowledge of the political climate for migrant workers in the United States.

However, I knew I couldn't run the research project without the time, labor, and political will of Filipino American youth in the grassroots organizations of the community. I was greatly concerned about the imposition I was placing on students who were juggling school and work, and young professionals had their own careers to look after. Two of the women who volunteered brought their small children to the kuwentuhan sessions. Still, we found ways to meet the various needs of the volunteers of the CARE Project. The ideas of inclusion came from the Filipino American youth who volunteered their time for our bayanihan effort. To name a few, we created a child-minding corner with volunteers to engage the children at the Filipino Community Center in order to allow mothers to participate in the kuwentuhan sessions. We figured out ways for students to include their CARE Project work in their senior theses and courses. After conducting kuwentuhan sessions, we would hold a debriefing session with volunteers, I was amazed at their ability to connect their own families' struggles to those of the care workers in our project. Additionally, their earnest curiosity and recognition of their own positionality and privilege became an apparent and valuable contribution to the process as a whole. Their technological dexterity, quick problem-solving skills, flexible schedules for setup or drop-off for the care workers, their willingness to sort out child care for the women activists in the room—all of these details that made the project run came from the cooperation and innovation of young people. In a *salamat* circle, or an ending discussion circle, where we expressed gratitude to a member of our research project who stood at the center of the circle, many workers expressed their thanks, or *pagsasalamat*, to the working professionals and young people in the room, and likewise, migrant workers were acknowledged for their bravery to share their story, their *kuwento*. The organic ways in which the community came together to support care workers sparked my thinking about just how these participatory processes and kuwentuhan itself could open up a portal for cultural understanding and political solidarity.

I continued to develop kuwentuhan and collaboration in other types of research projects that I took on following the CARE Project. In 2017 I led a research project on Filipino language access in San Francisco. I worked with a research group of undergraduate Filipina sociologists at SF State, training them in kuwentuhan. We collected kuwentuhan with ten service-providing organizations across San Francisco about the effects of not having access to city resources without translation and interpretation to the Filipino language. My students, or as I called them, co-researchers, and I discussed our kuwentuhan sessions, analyzed transcripts, came up with themes, and

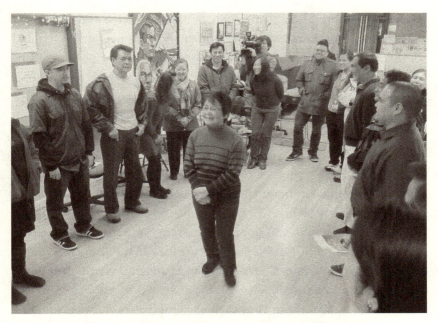

A caregiver stands in the middle of a *salamat* circle of community at the end of a session, 2012

presented and published our findings together.[1] Although this project was scaled back in many ways, kuwentuhan was the driving qualitative method for the group because it helped connect our Filipina research team to the Filipina/o service providers. While it wasn't fully participatory in nature, I believe my methodology was transformed by the original CARE Project in that I could not fathom conducting kuwentuhan work on issues plaguing the Filipino community without the collaboration of its young people. Even on a project about language access, it was clear that kuwentuhan as a method allowed for my students to step into their roles as researchers and, more important, conducting research that would benefit their Filipino community in San Francisco.

A few years later, in the midst of the global pandemic in 2020, a later iteration of the CARE Project—kuwentuhan sessions over Zoom—became the main method of my continued aims to support Filipino care workers and the migrant organizations that served them. Through a collaboration with PAWIS in the South Bay Area and Filipino American students at SF

State, we began to conduct kuwentuhan digitally to create space for care workers to communicate with one another and consult with lawyers and organizers about issues at their workplaces. Although Zoom might be commonplace now, four years into the COVID-19 pandemic, in mid-2020, it was still a new technology that we were all learning to use. When our kuwentuhan session's Zoom room opened up, the students on my research team would call the care workers on the roster to ensure they had the correct version of the app downloaded to their iPads, iPhones, and Androids. They would remain on the phone with care workers until cameras were unveiled and mute buttons were unmuted. Once these logistical items were squared away, the care workers had free rein over the space, and our kuwentuhan would last from one to two hours because the time to dialogue was so sorely needed by these invisible frontline workers. In the Zoom sessions, as caregivers shared their own issues living in a pandemic world, they would turn the conversation around to ask the students, "*Ikaw? Paano na ang school mo?* How about you? How's school going for you?" It was a mutual recognition that while the pandemic had different impacts on each of us, we all needed to say aloud the very things that were weighing heavily on our minds. During the debriefing sessions after the virtual kuwentuhan, students would comment about how powerful the conversations were and how they underestimated how much they, too, needed the time and space to process what life was like under the pandemic. In many ways, the topics of discussion in kuwentuhan were co-constructed by Filipino migrant workers, the Filipino American young people who participated, and myself. Each of us contributed to a robust conversation about experiencing the crisis from our individual perspectives. For care workers, their urgent needs were about their work conditions. For young people, they were witnessing how their families and households, chock-full of health-care workers, were affected by the pandemic. It was the collaboration among us that allowed for care workers to share their stories and, ultimately, spur organizing work toward their plight.

In both of these instances of my longitudinal relationship- and organization-building work with Filipino caregivers and Filipino American youth, it has been the method of kuwentuhan that has knitted us together to achieve a set of goals. Whether it was exposing the frequency of wage theft in the caregiving sector in San Francisco, calling attention to language access issues for Filipino newcomers, or swapping essential information about COVID-19, the first-, 1.5-, and second-generation Filipinas/os who participated in the projects to support migrants and migrant workers were creating an ethics of care that has become a guiding force and motivation in my academic and political work. Kuwentuhan as a method has been a container for many difficult conversations, but, most important, it has taught me how to hold people with care in all of their complex selves. It provides an altar to offer up our most challenging moments, our joys, and our simple pleasures. It is a way to commune with one another.

I am committed to a sustained discussion of this methodology because I believe it is important to lay bare the co-constructive processes of research and scholarly knowledge production as systematic and creative, planned and circuitous. I have found that writing about the logics of inquiry and the years-long practices of building research relationships always reveals the many individuals, organizations, and communities that have co-constructed the research questions, data collection processes, analyses, and theories of change that I propose in practice and in my academic writing. Many Filipina/o Americans have reflected on the complex project of social science methods, and I join them in this reflexive practice.[2] Moreover, I surrender these methods to you, reader, as a gift—mostly because I have received these gifts in tenfold through my commitments to building movements that insist on investing in the power of migrant workers. It is my hope that in this reflection and discussion, many other researchers and organizers can innovate participatory methodologies and knowledge production that serves communities first.

In this chapter, I reflect on the methods of the multiple phases of collecting qualitative research for this book spanning a decade in which I engaged kuwentuhan as my primary method of data collection. Over the years, the participatory projects I designed often held Filipina/o migrant workers—often first-generation immigrants—at the center of my research process. Yet, Filipina/o Americans—1.5- and second-generation immigrants—who were students, recent graduates, professionals, and community members, were key in the processes of data collection, analysis, and dissemination. In this chapter I will discuss in depth kuwentuhan as a social science research method and as a political organizing tool, a reflexive practice around migration and transnationalism, and a conscientizing process. I aim to demonstrate that kuwentuhan not only allows for the empowerment and leadership development of Filipina/o migrant workers but also that it can spark a politics of solidarity and organizing across generations.

Beyond a "methods" chapter, I argue that the intergenerational and participatory aspects of the multiple phases of caregiver research engendered a politics and ethics of care that spanned immigrant generations. Leah Lakshmi Piepzna-Samarasinha, a disability and transformative justice activist, poet, and writer, has written about care webs and care collectives within disabled communities. She insists that the reciprocal practices of support and mutual aid must also include nondisabled people, requiring those who do not experience the world as sick and disabled to take part in strengthening these webs and collectives.[3] Following this political insight, I apply this conceptual trend to the cross-generational participants in my Filipino American community in the San Francisco Bay Area. I hope to tease out both methodological and theoretical contributions to an ethos of care that pulls the intellectual and political conversations around the advancement of migrant workers' dignity away from migrant workers alone. I enjoin you to think through how the struggle for migrant workers' rights and dignity is a project of entanglement, of intergenerational dialogue, activism, bravery, and solidarity, of a shared potential of radical care.

A SHORT NOTE ON A LONG HISTORY: LABOR EXPORT AND FILIPINO AMERICANS

Scholars have established that the Philippines, as a migrant-sending state, has organized its efforts to manage migration of its citizens through a de facto labor export policy that began in the 1970s.[4] In the first instance, the practice of exporting Filipino citizens under the Ferdinand Marcos dictatorship was to accrue capital in a newly neoliberalizing global economy. In subsequent decades, however, the sophisticated recruitment and management of migrant exports has been consolidated into what Robyn Rodriguez calls a "labor brokerage state," with scaffolding policies, cultural apparatuses, and institutions to support and encourage the labor migration of upward of 10 percent of the Philippine population.[5] The brokerage of Filipino labor globally has continued to this very day, changing the Filipino diaspora from a temporary solution to assuage political conflict in the Philippines to a permanent fixture of Filipino life.

Filipino migration to the Americas, and particularly what is now the United States, began in the sixteenth century through the Spanish Manila Galleon Trades between the archipelago, Mexico, and Spain. Under US imperial logics of benevolent assimilation and colonization, Spain acquired the Philippines as a commonwealth in 1898, thus spurring a long subsequent history of labor migration to the United States. Dawn Bohulano Mabalon found that the early stages of induced migration of Filipinos in the 1920s to the 1930s were a response to the labor shortages in US agricultural and fishing industries on the Pacific front, including Hawai'i, California, and Alaska.[6] Through the late twentieth century, the reorganization of the global economy found Filipinos in the Philippines working in labor-intensive and -exploitative factories and into the 2010s shifting toward global service economies.[7] Parallel to the political economic shifts in the Philippines, Filipino migrant labor to the United States continued through professional occupations such as nursing and teaching and in occupations of servitude.[8]

Because of the long history of Filipino migration to the United States, it follows that generations of Filipinos who were born in the United States (referred to as Filipino Americans from this point on) navigated their presence in US society, while a migration stream of Filipinos continues. Migration scholars coined the terms "first-," "1.5-," and "second-generation" immigrants to distinguish immigrants and their posterity. Richard Alba writes, "For immigrants to the USA, the 'generation' served as a temporal gauge of immigrant-group assimilation, where 'generation' is the ancestral distance from the point of arrival in a society."[9] In what follows, it is important to note that we use "first-generation" immigrants as those who immigrated to the United States when they were over the age of eighteen. I use Ruben Rumbaut's term "1.5-generation" to refer to children who arrived in the States between the ages of six and twelve and "second-generation" for children of immigrants who were born in the United States.[10] The use of generations, in the contexts of migration and one's relationship to the points of arrival to the United States, becomes a source of intergenerational conflict and dissonance among Filipino Americans and Filipino immigrants within families and in the ethnic community. The disjunctures among Filipino Americans and Filipinos in the States are shaped by the contrasts between immigration generations and are compounded by the difference in age, the more formal definition of "generations."

Still, Filipino American scholars assert that across immigration generations, return migration and transnational behaviors can continue among first-, 1.5-, and second-generation immigrants, albeit different in frequency and consistency.[11] Even if such conflicts among these generations exist, Filipino sociologists argue that subsequent generations sustain remittance behaviors started by their first-generation immigrant predecessors, return to the Philippines for charity and advocacy work, and even return to directly invest in real estate and urban development in the Philippines.[12] These studies demonstrate that immigrants' aspirations and goals extend beyond American sociological theories of migrant assimilation that position their desires to incorporate into American society and leave the "old world" behind. While their incorporation to the American social order shapes Filipino immigrants and subsequent generations' daily lives, we can also accept that, intergenerationally, Filipino migrants and Filipino Americans stay connected to their homeland in multiple ways.

Here, I submit that because of the complex context of Filipino Americans and Filipino immigrants, their generational differences can produce differences and conflict among them, and yet transnational connectivity lasts beyond the first generation of immigrants. To this end, I offer my reflection on culturally responsive methodology in the time of coronavirus, and the purchase it might have for Filipina/o researchers conducting studies under conditions of severity and crisis, while recognizing the possibility and currency of radical care.

DEVELOPING KUWENTUHAN AS PRAXIS

Drawing from a Philippine cultural practice of storytelling that facilitates the exchange of essential and quotidian information among its participants, kuwentuhan allows for participants to pick up and expound on themes they deem important. In kuwentuhan, individual and collective experiences are intertwined based on the Filipino cultural practice of talk-story. The act is recurring in many Filipino social spaces, such as family gatherings and church fellowship, and is a linguistic practice based on *kapwa*, a Filipino cultural value that acknowledges an individual's identity as shared with the collective other.[13] In effect, kuwentuhan fulfills the need to understand oneself in context with other Filipinos, fulfilling a need to connect and belong to a greater collective. I have employed kuwentuhan in all of my research projects with Filipino domestic workers in New York City and the San Francisco Bay Area, fostering an environment where Filipino migrants can draw from a daily and cultural exercise and engage on the topics they care most about.[14] Yet, in the past I have not discussed in depth how this method has always necessitated an intergenerational cooperation from Filipinas/os who are born in the United States or came to the country as children. For this book, the plight of Filipina/o care workers were and are entangled with the multigenerational lives of Filipina/o Americans and Filipina/o immigrants who shared households, churches, workplaces, and community spaces—and, in fact, the very methods that collated the important narratives that are at the center of this book. Kuwentuhan spans multiple generations of Filipino American community, generations in terms of age cohorts and in terms of immigrant cohorts. To this end, I argue that kuwentuhan, and other methods developed to reflect the social realities and epistemologies of participants, can not only advance social science research but it can also create space in community for dialogue, solidarity, and activism.

In 2009, when I was conducting research for my dissertation, which later became my book *The Labor of Care*, I had been trained in graduate school in social scientific qualitative methods such as ethnography, interviews, focus groups, participant observation, and content analysis, among others. In a complementary path, I was trained by my community organizing circles to listen carefully to members in our Filipino neighborhood in New York City so that we could understand and act on the issues they deemed urgent. These issues included labor exploitation, human trafficking, and unstable immigration statuses for many of the Filipino newcomers in Queens. As a doctoral student and a Filipina American, who was formerly undocumented and balancing the privilege with which I grew up as a young person in the United States, I held my identities as immigrant and American-raised in tension. I was also at the intersection of advanced social science training and my community's invitation to take my formal education and apply it to the needs of the Filipino immigrant community in New York. In many ways I still stand at this intersection, holding this generative, and often complicated, tension between Filipina and Filipina American, scholar and activist.

Fortunately, in graduate school I learned about the potentials and pitfalls of participatory action research (PAR) from education researchers in New York City and queer and disabled researchers of color.[15] What spoke to me about PAR as a methodology was flipping the script on who social scientists have erstwhile labeled "informants" or "research subjects" as active leaders and decision makers in the research process about their lives and communities. Rather than passive people whom research is being done "on," PAR had the potential to reverse the sedimentation of research participants to static beings in a research project. Instead, PAR could move participants to the center of research projects, directing the process and ethics of the work. From Black and Brown people working to protect their neighborhoods, ethnic studies students and teachers, young people in schools, and inmates and prisoners, I had many examples wherein PAR as a methodology could be a collaborative space for knowledge production and, more important, organizing for action and change.[16] PAR also demonstrated that different groups of people with different stakes in an issue could work together to produce projects and knowledge that could empower communities to seek justice and change.

The convergence of critical and feminist research methods and my transnational political organizing with the Philippine National Democratic movement from the United States challenged me to explore what participatory method(s) could look like in my work with Filipino migrant workers. While on a trip to integrate social movement organizations in the Philippines with GABRIELA and BAYAN Philippines, I was introduced to how activists rely on PAR in upland farming communities, among other sectors, to involve them in an educational process to uncover the need to organize and mobilize for basic needs and land reform. I got my hands on a printed copy of the *IBON Manual on Facilitating Participatory Research*. The

IBON Foundation is an independent research institute and databank, and in this manual they argue, "Research, like science, is only relevant when it is used for the welfare of the majority. It is important that research supports the social issues that need to be addressed because it provides the basis of a systematic, objective[,] resourceful and determined plan of action."[17] My weeks-long integration with female peasant communities in the upland farming region of Kalinga, in the northern Philippines, demonstrated that PAR could rely on indigenous people's everyday skills and inherited practices of keeping healthy relationships with the land. In fact, through PAR, indigenous people in Kalinga recognized that their long-established, self-reliant methods of farming could be the basis of advancing technologies that wouldn't rob their land of nutrients. In practice, I observed how PAR could engender trust between communities, activist researchers, and diasporic activists like myself. I felt excited about the possibility of democratizing research in service of the Filipino community in New York, basing my research on the objectives of people's organizations, especially those who worked with and for the interest of migrant workers, many of whom were working in sectors like domestic work and caregiving, just outside the purview of the formal labor unions. My logic was that, through PAR, not only could research processes produce data that could drive winnable campaigns to improve immigrant workers' work conditions, but that participatory process could also engage migrant workers in building relationships of trust and camaraderie among one another and with people who shared a commitment to building solidarity and power for migrant workers.

Generally, however, studies published on PAR in immigrant communities at the time deployed participatory methods to gain access to "hard-to-reach" immigrant populations where barriers of language and location kept immigrant communities isolated from researchers who did not come from the same communities.[18] PAR projects with immigrant communities were concerned with immigrants' health promotion, assessment of healthcare needs, and culturally relevant services. Some studies examine how immigrants and refugees sustain their participation in community-based participatory projects and the importance of immigrants' ethnocultural, contextual knowledge in collecting rich data on health outcomes.[19] In these studies, scholars made an auxiliary finding: engaging immigrants in PAR methods not only yields data for the community's health needs but also an increased sense of empowerment and health-promoting practices within the community.[20] While these studies employed PAR as a recruitment strategy on topics of utmost importance, I knew that my positionality as an immigrant, scholar, and activist could effectively change the dynamics of how I conducted PAR.

Recently, a special edition of an academic journal called *Migration Letters* featured PAR methods with migrants and migrant workers and the potential of the methodology to advance social justice issues focusing on the lives and experiences of migrants.[21] Still, scholars remind us that PAR is not the great equalizer—its potential to "empower" migrants or research participants can be trifled without researchers' cultural humility.[22] The allure of "empowerment" in PAR must be sobered by the longitudinal process of research and the protracted evolution of conscientization, political organizing, and movement building. Rather than PAR as an outreach tool or a process to find a moment of empowerment, it is my experience that the subjectivities and experiences of im/migrants in and of itself amid the research process can be valuable for political organizing, research analysis, and development of action strategies. Methods of PAR allow migrants to reflect on the very systems of power that have contributed to creating their experiences of migration.

In my record of conducting and writing about PAR with Filipino migrants for a decade and a half, I have found that workers have a deep understanding of institutionalized labor export and therefore are undoubtedly experts in the mechanisms and experiences of induced migration.[23] Participatory data collection, data analysis, and dissemination of findings (in various outcomes, events, and products) create possibilities for migrants to reflect on their experiences and draw out their systemic analyses of how they came to the United States. Migrants often try to make sense of their migration experiences (e.g., long-term separation, difficulties in transitioning to destination countries, etc.) through their immigrant social networks and daily talk-stories.[24] The collective approach to participatory methods can echo those very transnational cultural practices of Filipinos who value belonging to a larger community (of Filipinos, immigrants, transnational persons).[25]

I learned from Hawai'ian and indigenous researchers and scholars who designed methodology to use talk-story, a cultural style of communication and meaning making, for projects that lifted up indigenous voices toward action and change.[26] With PAR as a methodology—that is, a logic of inquiry, not a prescribed set of methods from which communities are then invited to participate in—there was a need and a basis to explore developing kuwentuhan to mirror the collectivist nature of participatory research. Over chatter-filled Sunday dinners or group subway rides in New York City, it was clear that Filipina/o migrant workers were already engaging in the important social scientific processes of analyzing their new environs, New York City. Philippine studies scholars had long discussed *pakikipagkuwentuhan* as a method of collecting qualitative experiences about Filipinos' personal and collective experiences.[27] Similar to the native Hawai'ian talk-story, where the discussions among community members were key in making meaning and achieving a sense of relationality to one another, a core way of indigenous people's understanding of self, there were many ways I had observed this dynamic in the community organizing work I was doing. After all, the Filipino value of kapwa, where one shared their identity with another, was established through trading stories and exchanging lessons in an informal discussion in social spaces.

When I first began my collaboration with Filipina/o domestic workers in New York City, many of them felt nervous or too shy to participate in a research project that collected interviews when I spoke about it in those terms. Reflecting on those words, to this day I can say that many Filipinos attach the ideas of research to institutional and authoritative entities such as universities and government agencies, by which they have felt harmed and tokenized. Ultimately, they count themselves out of "those" who produce knowledge and create theories of change. Yet the types of mutual aid, feminist and interracial solidarity, and organic intellectualism I have seen and experienced in migrant worker organizing circles have been rich wells of political theory for political struggle. And much of the innovative strategies for building community and creating conditions for action often took place in kuwentuhan over a plate of food and loud karaoke. So asking domestic workers to engage in kuwentuhan rather than "interviews" immediately put their apprehension at ease and tapped into their daily cultural practice of kuwento as a form of fostering trust and relationships through the exchange of experiences.

A few years and many institutional moves later, in the San Francisco Bay Area, when I started a new project with domestic workers, I, along with a group of migrant worker leaders and 1.5- and second-generation community members, came to an agreement about conducting research together. We would all participate in crafting the research topics, constructing guides with themes we believed were important to migrant workers, learning how kuwentuhan could be a source of knowledge production in our community, then conducting kuwentuhan and analyzing its content. In these formative beginning phases, kuwentuhan became a reliable recruitment method for migrant workers for sharing their stories, no matter how traumatic or uneventful they were. For migrant workers, kuwentuhan was already a practice that informed their daily exchanges. They felt like experts in it—for them, learning and wielding the method under the mode of research was second nature. For me, it pushed me to think creatively about my positionality as a scholar and activist and, more important, what it meant to democratize research and scholarship, research processes and outcomes. While the intellectual and academic questions and projects were what I needed to advance my intellectual body of work, the more urgent political questions were where I believed I could best contribute my scholarly training. Thus, the undergirding motivation of creating kuwentuhan as a method was, How will research or scientific investigation of the lives of Filipino migrant workers contribute to political change and power in their hands?

INTERGENERATIONAL METHODOLOGY

Though I've written about the power of PAR in building migrant worker power, I have yet to explore deeply the role of 1.5- and second-generation Filipina/o Americans in all of the PAR projects I've collaborated on. It was only in 2022 with, at the time, doctoral student Edwin Carlos that I explored the impacts of kuwentuhan with migrant workers on the young people and students who provide essential support on PAR projects.[28] It was through the cowriting and conversations with Edwin that this chapter came to being. Although I do not have the copious amounts of qualitative data on the experiences of the Filipina/o Americans during these projects that they do (rightfully so, given they were not the focus of the projects), their voices are in a majority of the kuwentuhan sessions as notetakers and tech troubleshooters. Their presence during the creative and academic processes to produce different outcomes is unbroken. In the PAR projects I helped to lead with the migrant worker organizations MIGRANTE NYC and GABRIELA NYC between 2008 and 2010, and MIGRANTE San Francisco between 2011 and 2012, the roles of students, young people, and Filipina/o Americans as collaborators, tech support, resource finders, creative partners, carpoolers, meal preparers, intellectual companions, organizing allies, and change makers have been regrettably understated in my work. During the collection phases for this book in 2017–2018 and then again in 2020, the projects I deem "PAR lite," it was the work and commitment of Filipina/o Americans that helped me achieve and democratize the research process. So in what follows, I want to trace how the development of kuwentuhan began with the organic intellectualism of migrant workers and to theorize its purchase on intergenerational understanding and activism.

As I have stated in other parts of this book, the evidence used for my theorization here had many starts and stops. Finishing up my dissertation as a fellow at the University of San Francisco in 2011, the need for a research project was initiated by the Filipino Community Center Workers' Rights Program coordinator, Mario de Mira, who noticed that so many Filipino migrants were affected by the same issue: *wage theft*, a term that describes how employers withhold pay from migrant workers based on a range of deductions that may not be legal.[29] The Filipino Community Center organizers wanted to engage in a systematic investigation of how common this problem was. I, along with Dr. Robyn Rodriguez and University of California, Davis, GABRIELA San Francisco members, Filipino American students from SF State and University of San Francisco, teamed up with Filipino Community Center worker leaders to create a PAR program that echoed the process in New York City.

An intergenerational group of community members, migrant workers, students, and academics, we all engaged in research training and participatory data collection through kuwentuhan and then produced a fact sheet and cultural theater piece based on the narratives we collected. In this project, the workers' rights program needed data on just how widespread the issue of wage theft was; we were also interested in organizing migrant workers through the process of exchanging stories and uncovering problematic issues that workers might have in common. In addition, the center wanted to work on creating a cultural theatrical production to present a composite story of Filipino migrant workers' lives. The various organizations and academics involved were invested in supporting migrant workers in building collective power and creating opportunities for second-generation Filipino Americans to learn the pressing issues migrant workers faced. This second objective was not fully in focus for our project, but since many of the Filipina/o Americans who signed up to be part of the project were part of campus or grassroots organizations, I proposed that their participation in the CARE Project could be political education and increased awareness of the issues and experiences of Filipino migrant workers. Just as a young activist I learned about the social realities of workers and peasants and their movement strategies in the Philippines, the young people involved in the PAR project learned about the conditions of Filipino migrant workers in their very backyard while participating in discovering solutions for those issues.

My original plan for this book was a 2017 mixed-methods study called the CARE Project at San Francisco State University that examined stress levels among Filipino caregivers in the San Francisco Bay Area. The study used a quantitative survey measuring mental health outcomes for caregivers and kuwentuhan after participants took the survey.[30] The 2017–2018 survey was supposed to be a springboard for a PAR project that would invite Filipino care workers to be trained in kuwentuhan and engage them in a collaborative effort of collecting data. Alongside Filipino migrant organizers, we were collaborating on crafting methods that heeded a "culture-centered approach" to examine the health outcomes of migrant care workers that could examine the structural determinants and health behaviors of migrants.[31] As I have done in the past, I planned on engaging PAR methodology and principles because doing so would allow for migrants and migrant workers to assert their lived experiences as "expertise." After the survey and kuwentuhan were completed, I would bring back the major themes to the worker organizations I collaborated with so that we could think through how PAR methods could not only help prioritize the organizing campaigns of worker organizations but also how they could become useful for ongoing

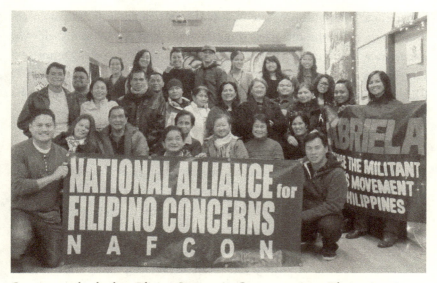

Caregiver worker leaders, Filipino Community Center organizers, Filipinx American students, Filipinx American women from GABRIELA San Francisco, and members of National Alliance for Filipino Concerns celebrate a kuwentuhan session, 2012

research and leadership development for migrant worker leaders. In 2017 I also had my second child, a baby boy named Cy Andres. While I juggled an infant, a tenure-track job, community involvement, and this research project, I necessarily took a slower pace in carrying out the research process.

Still, I believed that PAR methods could assist with building up migrant worker leaders, and thus migrant worker organizations, because the process and method draw from the social realities of migrant workers' experiences of migration and domestic labor.[32] For example, while migrants and their decisions to migrate are constrained by the Philippine state and the global economy, the state often labels them as aloof or incompetent workers if problems of abuse or exploitation occur when they are working abroad. Migrant workers often blame themselves for their inability to protect or defend themselves from exploitation, wage theft, and abuse. However, in my work I have demonstrated that kuwentuhan captures migrants' individual narratives as it is situated in the production of migrants as exports because when their stories are collected and analyzed by peers, they are able to see that their individual experiences of hardship are actually a collective experience.[33] The political potential in kuwentuhan and participatory research processes presents itself when migrant workers recount their own experiences and begin to understand that individual stories comprise a larger story of forced migration, labor export policy, and low-wage work.[34] This micro-macro resonance in PAR is why I invest in kuwentuhan as a culturally responsive logic of inquiry for Filipino migrants.

In 2019, student researchers Elaika Celemen, Kristal Osorio, and I analyzed the data from the survey and published preliminary findings arguing that the crisis for caregivers relied on normalizing exploitation in their workplaces.[35] At this time, I was planning how to outreach to Filipino care workers and establish relationships with Filipino migrant worker organizations in the Bay Area to develop a PAR project that might yield both intellectual and political gains for my community. In early 2020, however, COVID-19 changed everything. My visions of training a new cadre of caregivers in research processes and leadership development were hampered with the changes of lockdown. Care workers themselves were navigating an entirely new world of quarantine, PPE, or the lack thereof, and coronavirus—still working and quite unprepared. My research plans would have to either wait or adapt.

A year before the onset of the pandemic, the Filipinx Count! survey was launched by the UC Davis Bulosan Center for Filipinx Studies, the first center in the country devoted to the study of Filipinx Americans. The survey data questions included topics such as health, immigration, employment, mental and physical health, and access to health care. I partnered with the Bulosan Center and in collaboration with PAWIS in Silicon Valley to use kuwentuhan as a form of collecting stories to understand the experiences of caregivers under COVID-19. Along with Dr. Robyn Rodriguez, doctoral student and, at the time, research director, R. J. Taggueg, in consultation with PAWIS worker leader Tess Brillante and Felwina Mondina, I proposed that we continue using a revised version of the Filipinx Count! survey to monitor how Filipino care workers were faring in the pandemic. It would also serve as a way for organizations and scholar-activists to continue to meet with care workers online during shelter-in-place.

An innovative aspect of this PAR project was in the methodological choice to not only involve first-generation immigrants working as care workers but to also include 1.5- and second-generation students as co-researchers in the participatory research processes. By living and conducting research in the San Francisco Bay Area, which has a high concentration of Filipina/o immigrants, I knew that working with Filipina/o American students and young people would inevitably include their family and community members who work in the caregiving industry. While we recruited participants through multiple avenues—such as partnerships with Filipino-serving community-based organizations, Filipino American events, and families of 1.5- and second-generation Filipina/o Americans—the decision to include those students and youth as co-researchers also gave the study an intergenerational exploratory component as to how multigenerational households and families were dealing with the pandemic.

Participatory research processes with first-, 1.5-, and second-generation immigrants included recruitment of Filipino and care workers, training to lead logistics of kuwentuhan sessions via Zoom to collect the experiences of Filipino care workers, qualitative data training and analysis, and, lastly, the synthesis and presentation of findings to academic and community audiences. In this effort, I organized and trained a group of eight 1.5- and second-generation undergraduate and graduate students to work on the research team, along with three first-generation caregiver immigrants working as participatory advisors and co-researchers.

Initially, the research questions of this study revolved around the work conditions and well-being of Filipino care workers. However, during the pandemic the care workers I *would have* recruited and engaged in a fully participatory research process were inundated with new and unprecedented changes in their workplaces. Their adjustments to lockdowns and online formats of meeting and organizing was a steep learning curve. To say that Filipino caregivers were overwhelmed is an understatement. The participation of 1.5- and second-generation co-researchers who were also the children and relatives of Filipino caregivers became a bridge for the digital divides of Zoom meetings as the main form of qualitative data collection. The technological dexterity of 1.5- and second-generation young people facilitated the Zoom kuwentuhans and the creation of infographics to disseminate the findings of the study.

All co-researchers in the CARE Project, a total of eight people, represented a range of immigrants from the first, 1.5, and second generations and had varying relationships to Filipinos working in the care industry, which produced anticipated findings about the work conditions of care workers under the COVID-19 pandemic but also unanticipated findings about intergenerational understanding among immigrant cohorts. The student researchers I worked with were undergraduates as well as newly graduated and graduate students: Alyssa Barquin, Elaika Celemen, Chloe Punsalan, Renee Zapata, Tanya Yared, Edwin Carlos, Katherine Nasol, and R. J. Taggueg at San Francisco State University, University of California, Berkeley, and University of California, Davis.

As 1.5- and second-generation co-researchers helped facilitate technology and ensured that notes were taken during virtual kuwentuhan sessions, first-generation care workers led the Zoom discussions. During the hours-long conversations on Zoom, student researchers who are either immigrants themselves or children of first-generation immigrants were moved by the difficult situations described in the testimonies of care workers. In our debrief sessions, 1.5- and second-generation co-researchers reflected what they heard in "their parents' and grandparents'" stories in the experiences shared during the data collection. Co-researchers from the 1.5- and second-generations whose relatives participated in the study commented that the experience of being present during the interview or kuwentuhan or transcribing and coding the data from their relatives helped them discover intimate parts of their own family's story that they would have not been privy to if it weren't for the research project.[36] They went on to say that even if their parents or grandparents weren't care workers, they learned the humanity in the struggle that their elders went through as they were striving to make a life in United States.

A key unanticipated finding of having first-, 1.5-, and second-generation co-researchers participating in the study was the transnational critique that became embedded in many of our analysis sessions. While first-generation immigrants could clearly articulate the problems in the Philippines that induced their migrations, 1.5- and second-generation co-researchers were twice removed from those realities because they had either moved to the United States as children or were born here. In conducting research that included the stories of first-generation migrants' lives in the Philippines, however, 1.5- and second-generation co-researchers could quickly ascertain the structural lack of jobs and livelihood in the Philippines that push Filipinos to migrate. More important, 1.5- and second-generation co-researchers could identify why so many Filipino care workers in the United States had to grit their teeth through stories of the exploitation and abuse that were shared during the kuwentuhan sessions. Although the transnational connections of 1.5- and second-generation co-researchers consisted of the relationships their parents or relatives developed for them, their participation in this study opened the opportunity for them to understand their positionality to the Philippines' labor export policy and its generational impacts abroad.

KUWENTUHAN AS A PORTAL FOR INTERGENERATIONAL UNDERSTANDING

Migration studies scholars agree that PAR is a useful methodology in understanding migration and transnationalism.[37] Migration scholars using PAR have argued that its methodological potential for innovation contributes to a robust understanding of migrants' experiences and, possibly, transformation of their social conditions.[38] Elsewhere I have argued that including the role of migrants in PAR should not serve simply as a method to access hard-to-reach contacts; rather, it can be a process to develop methods to draw out migrant expertise.[39] While the burgeoning literature on PAR methodologies in migrant communities is promising, often the participation of migrants has included just one generation. Some PAR studies have engaged young migrants and children of migrants, but those studies often engage young people's relationship to the assimilative pressures in their new destination countries.[40] Yet as I have shown, kuwentuhan, as developed in my past PAR projects, has demonstrated that intergenerational cooperation among first-, 1.5-, and second-generation migrants can play a major role in developing our academic and political understanding of experiences of migration and transnationalism. In kuwentuhan the exchange of individual stories and the emergence of a collective story can be a salve for migrants who have experienced similar struggles. Moreover, the process can also yield robust and critical knowledge consisting of migrants' lived experiences as "expertise" about the global institutionalization of migration and low-wage migrant work in the United States. For Filipina/o Americans, who do not share the lived experience of labor migration, kuwentuhan can produce critical questions and discussions that ultimately lead to conscientization around the plight of migrant workers. More important, for 1.5- and second-generation Filipina/o Americans, being involved in kuwentuhan allows them an exploration of experiences that are adjacent to their own families' stories. I now turn to how kuwentuhan in PAR projects can encourage an exploration of transnational connectivity between 1.5- and second-generation migrant youth and the experiences of first-generation people in their community.

Defining Intergenerational and Intragenerational

I use "*inter*generational dialogue" to describe the conversations and interactions among different generations of migrants, such as between first-generation migrants and second-generation children of immigrants born in the United States. "*Intra*generational dialogue" describes conversations within a particular ethnic immigrant group—in this study, Filipinos in the United States. I point to inter- and intragenerational dialogue to think through the co-construction of narratives and stories about Filipinos' lived experiences as a methodological innovation in the participatory process. I argue that conducting PAR during the pandemic necessitated avenues of participation outside of the "subjects" of the research project—first-generation Filipina/o care workers. Rather, the inter- and intragenerational dialogue of kuwentuhan, which became our primary research method, facilitated an understanding of migration and transnationalism involving first-generation Filipina/o care workers *and* 1.5- and second-generation co-researchers in the study.

As 1.5- and second-generation co-researchers used inter- and intragenerational kuwentuhan, they too came to some understanding about their liminality in living in the United States and their own connections transnationally. Inter- and intragenerational kuwentuhan about migration and transnationalism emphasizes how migration is not an event but instead an experiential process that affects how these people understand their family, story, and identity. For Filipina/o Americans, the practice of kuwentuhan happens regularly in dialogue among family members, peers, and researchers with their interviewees. I describe different aspects of dialogue and interactions between and within generations of migrant communities, most from Filipino contexts, that situate why inter- and intragenerational dialogue, or kuwentuhan, is an invaluable innovation for the PAR projects described in this book.

Intergenerational Dialogue

Scholars argue that first-generation migrants pass down their transnational practices and activities to their children, second-generation immigrants, through their family lives.[41] Armand Gutierrez argues that 1.5- and second-generation Filipino Americans who engage in "mediated social and economic cross-border ties collectively with their first-generation migrant parents" learn about and perpetuate their transnational ties through this mediated relationship between their parents and nonmigrant recipients in the Philippines.[42] Filipino Americans thus feel a filial obligation to parents who ask that their children engage in transnational social and economic ties. The decision to not send economic support to nonmigrant recipients in the Philippines is also mediated by first-generation migrant parents, as 1.5- and second-generation children often stopped sending money home when parents severed ties or discouraged their children from remitting. Without first-generation parents bridging and encouraging transnational connections, it is likely that second-generation children disengage from transnational social and economic ties.

Indeed, studies show that second-generation immigrants continue transnational connections as a learned practice in their families depending on how the first-generation migrant parents decide to engage with the home country.[43] Additionally, second-generation immigrants sustain not only social and economic ties but also political ties that include interest and investment in the political situation in the home country even as they participate in the countries that receive them.[44] Filipino Americans of the 1.5 and second generations learn about the sociopolitical situation of the Philippines through the experience of first-generation immigrants and nonmigrants in the Philippines, particularly in issues involving migrant workers and natural disasters like Typhoon Haiyan in 2013.[45] The interest in engaging and helping these situations persists as 1.5- and second-generation migrants comprehend the role they can play while they are in the United States. This learning creates a connection with the Philippines that lends itself to more conversation with first-generation immigrant parents. Yet 1.5- and second-generation immigrants' transnational practices are quite different from first-generation immigrants. For example, second-generation migrants do not remit funds as frequently as their parents, and first-generation immigrants have established connections between the 1.5- and second-generation children and the homeland that may persist or shift, depending on conversations with their first-generation immigrant parents.[46]

Intragenerational Dialogue in Filipino Communities

Still, not all dialogue across immigrant generations—even in the same ethnic group, such as Filipinos—proves to be productive in transmitting beliefs between an older and younger generation. At times, rifts can be troubling between immigrant parents and their children, especially in terms of gender, wherein boys are allowed particular privileges that girls are not.[47] These rifts may make conversations intergenerationally more difficult and strained, thus necessitating more intragenerational dialogue among 1.5- and second-generation children to understand and garner support regarding these difficulties of this generational rift.

Scholars have argued that the marginalization that 1.5- and second-generation Filipino Americans experience in education is shaped by their parents' immigration and transnational experiences and the opportunities that 1.5- and second-generation Filipino Americans must understand from their parents' experiences.[48] Goals for higher education for second-generation migrants and their first-generation parents can sometimes compete with other goals for upward mobility. Scholars have argued that education assists in "upward" assimilation for second-generation immigrants into a white American middle-class conception, and although this may be a goal of first-generation parents for their children, cultural disconnects can occur because of this attempted upward assimilation.[49] For those who can draw on strong ethnic attachments and understanding in their migrant communities, moreover, 1.5- and second-generation immigrants' positive outlooks on schooling can be influenced by identity-based organizations or "cultural portals" that engage in dialogue surrounding their identity to make sense of liminal situations as Filipino Americans.[50] Indeed, having Filipino friends or mentors, participating in ethnic identity workshops, attending Filipino studies and language courses, and joining Filipino organizations can serve as spaces for intragenerational dialogue that contextualize what it means to be Filipino, American, and Filipino American through various conversations relating to culture, history, politics, and family.[51] These conversations serve to provide context for the goals of upward mobility that first-generation migrant parents often have for their children, allowing young people to co-construct their own identities in conversation with one another.

Family dynamics and generational differences, informed by cultural differences and upbringing, can result in a lack of communication between immigrant generations in the same ethnic groups, making intragenerational dialogue between first-, 1.5-, and second-generation migrants necessary. This lack of conversation can complicate the experience of 1.5- and second-generation immigrants as they negotiate their subjecthood in the United States as transnational subjects, even though their first-generation migrant parents may be the ones most directly affected by transnationalism.[52] Yet evidence has demonstrated that acknowledging the validity and specificity of struggles of each immigrant generation can produce an understanding between the two generations.[53] This acknowledgment of validity and specificity can happen intragenerationally between 1.5- and second-generation people, allowing for the co-construction of what it means to be transnational subjects in relation to their understandings of their first-generation parents' experiences.

In fact, I argue that if transnational practices between and among first-, 1.5-, and second-generation immigrants can be explored, it might be useful in producing the types of understanding that could bridge understanding between first-generation migrants and subsequent generations. The transnational experience is constantly co-constructed in conversations intergenerationally and intragenerationally, and the ways that one participates in transnational connections continues to grow. The use of kuwentuhan can open methodological opportunities to foster dialogue across generations within immigrant communities. First-, 1.5-, and second-generation immigrants may seldom have the space for dialogue and reconciliation specifically because of the assumption that assimilation trumps transnationalism. When it is quite the opposite, in the projects that I have conducted, 1.5- and second-generation immigrants have volunteered in droves to learn about the issues that newcomers and migrant workers experience as they arrive and adjust to life in the United States. Without overstating this fact, I believe that engaging in PAR projects and organizing campaigns to support migrant worker leadership and power can introduce these immigrants to new practices of transnationalism rooted in local political organizing efforts and transnational and intergenerational activism that is critical of the Philippine labor export system and global neoliberalism.

THE POTENTIAL OF KUWENTUHAN

In conducting kuwentuhan through PAR processes, I learned and I argue that this method and participatory methodology can produce inter-and intragenerational understanding among co-ethnics of different immigrant generations. In past studies, I found that through kuwentuhan the PAR process validated the experiences of Filipino first-generation care workers, thereby allowing migrant workers to build a critical solidarity with one another.[54] The process of collecting and listening to one another's work conditions allowed first-generation care workers to gain an understanding that conditions of exploitation and abuse was not an indicator of individual failure on their part but a symptom of a structurally inequitable industry of care work in the United States. When 1.5- and second-generation immigrants participate in kuwentuhan, they also bear witness to the individual testimonies of migrant workers and the class consciousness–building happening through their conversations and subsequent organizing. For the 1.5- and second-generation co-researchers, the participatory research process assisted with deeper understanding of the immigrant narratives that were anchored in the data we collected but also drew from their own familial experiences of migration and transnationalism. Often, one sociological assumption of 1.5- and second-generation immigrant youth is that they have more opportunities to advance in American society, even if there are structural disadvantages based on socioeconomic status, race, ethnicity, language, and cultural capital. However, the co-researchers from these generations across my projects attested to the fact that discovering one's own transnational identity is as important as understanding one's structural positionality in American society.

Philippine studies scholars have asserted that *pakikipagkuwentuhan*—or the daily practice of storytelling—is a low-stakes communicative engagement, which can include quotidian issues or sensitive, deeply personal issues.[55] At times, questions about the stress and difficulties of immigrant newcomer experiences are too difficult to discuss with one's own parents or grandparents. Often, the future orientation of first-generation Filipino immigrants can prevent them from sharing just how grueling it was to start and sustain a life in the United States. However, when 1.5- and second-generation co-researchers could listen to and witness the exchanges between the migrant workers in our kuwentuhan sessions, they were able to reflect on their own families' immigration experiences. Kuwentuhan, albeit adjacent to their own families' experiences, became a dialogue where immigrants were encouraged to speak about *and listen* to the experiences of adjustment to American life. While second-generation Filipina/o Americans are crafting their activism through rest, art, dance, joy, and song, a reimaging of the Filipino American archive, gender-expansive praxis and theorization, pedagogy and teaching, mutual aid and activist networks, and beyond, kuwentuhan can be one way that such activism is generated and sustained.[56]

With kuwentuhan as the main method, 1.5- and second-generation immigrant co-researchers not only gained a perspective on their own family's histories, but they were also encouraged to show up as allies to migrant workers who were organizing and developing their own leadership in their organizations. In the different versions of the CARE Project, first-generation Filipina/o migrant worker leaders often realized that 1.5- and second-generation immigrant co-researchers were genuinely interested to learn about their stories and wanted to engage them about the pressing issues migrant workers faced. For example, 1.5- and second-generation immigrant co-researchers volunteered during organizational drives for PPE and online social events. Many of the young people in the research projects that spanned a decade became deeply involved in community organizations that prioritized services for Filipino migrants in terms of housing, food security, labor rights, public health, and immigration law. In this way, kuwentuhan was not only a moment of data collection; it was also a point of entry toward mobilization and solidarity among first-generation migrant workers, a beginning process to galvanize solidarity across generations in the Filipino American community.

CONCLUSION

Reframing how I write about the participatory research projects for this book as intergenerational first-, 1.5-, and second-generation Filipina/o immigrants as research collaborators allowed an opening for intergenerational understanding through the intragenerational dialogue through kuwentuhan. Co-researchers from the 1.5 and second generations reported that the data collection process indirectly helped them to connect their own families' histories of migration and transnationalism to the experiences of first-generation migrants in the broader Filipino community. We learned that 1.5- and second-generation young people have important insights about migration that are not captured in the story of transnationalism because they are removed from the point of arrival. And in this study, in fact, 1.5- and second-generation young people taught us that migration is not an event; rather, immigration is a lifelong and sustained multigenerational process. We can turn to 1.5- and second-generation youth to provide deep insight as to how dialogue within and between immigrant generations can enable deeper understanding of the struggles and resilience within a migrant community.

Indeed, understanding the value of intergenerational and intragenerational dialogue in the PAR process allows for a deeper analysis of 1.5- and second-generation migrants as transnational beings. The development of transnational practices, sense of identity, and understandings of the historical and political contexts happens continuously in dialogues between and within migrant generations, and kuwentuhan allows these conversations to

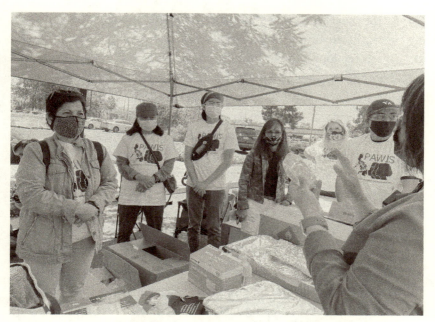

Caregiver worker leaders and Filipinx American youth gather during a protective personal equipment drive organized by PAWIS in Milpitas, 2021

be co-constructed. Indeed, using kuwentuhan as a method to understand transnational experiences with those being interviewed and the researchers in the study allows for a co-construction of the transnational identity for current and future generations.

Through participatory methodology and kuwentuhan, the possibilities for solidarity, advocacy, and political organization across migrant generational cohorts are plenty. I echo Caitlin Cahill's statement: "Working with rather than *for* PAR is a commitment to collaboration in its most profound sense as not only a politics of engagement but of solidarity."[57] Filipina/o Americans, both 1.5- and second-generation, exercised a solidarity with first-generation migrant working-class Filipinos, some of whom are their parents, relatives, and community members. In fact, kuwentuhan allowed us to build a "community of care" especially under a pandemic that began with sharing virtual space and making room for experiences offered through kuwento.[58] Lastly, while these communities of care already existed in the Filipino community, an explicit PAR process can build bonds between immigrant generations that stimulate sustainable solidarity and organizing efforts. In the future, I encourage scholars, activists, researchers, and teachers to try kuwentuhan in their projects and spaces and explore its potentials and limitations. I invite you to think about kuwentuhan as part of a critical Filipinx American studies collective commons—to document and analyze, to innovate and expand. Many already are.[59]

I want to end on a personal note. It was Celine Parreñas Shimizu who provoked me gently, in a public forum about *The Labor of Care*, about how I would sustain such intensely participatory methods in my upcoming research projects. After all, in 2018, when my first book was published and when the forum occurred, I had two children under four years old buzzing around. Immediately, I had no clue. Sleep-deprived and on tenure track, I had no idea how I would continue PAR moving forward, as it is a time-intensive effort. But it was my children, Aya and Cy, both second-generation Filipina/o Americans, who taught me that the goal of an ethic of care in scholar-activism, in developing methods to bolster movement building, is necessary. Aya and Cy, and the time limitations that come with raising a family as an academic, showed me that passing the methodology—that is, the logic of inquiry and the logic *for* action—on to future generations is key in redefining kuwentuhan as a method and praxis.

EPILOGUE

I often think about the different versions of myself that I've offered up to you in this book: my ten-year-old new immigrant eyes learning my grandmother's routine at the care home; a mother juggling teaching, research, and raising two small children under a global pandemic; a scholar-activist figuring out the riddle of creating meaningful research in service of my communities. I reflect on these phases in my life knowing one thing is sure: it was the love and commitment of loved ones that helped shape my ethics of care. In this book, I began by framing the stories of Filipino caregivers with the theories of social reproductive labor and racial capitalism, aimed at contextualizing the invisibility of caregivers and the care crisis in the contradictions of late-stage capitalism. My effort in going on to elucidate the constant and relentless work conditions of caregivers as a normalized environment for long-term care was meant to demonstrate that indeed the work of caregivers is skilled and encumbered by the lack of political imagination and will for the aging population and their care workers in the United States. In some instances, writing about the lives of caregivers working during the COVID-19 pandemic was a necessary moment to shed light on just how essential care workers are to our society and that perhaps it is in our relationships and dialogue with younger generations that a culture centering on the necessity of care and recognizing the labor it requires can change our world. The work and activism of Filipino care workers has shaped me from my childhood to my motherhood.

One of my clearest memories as an immigrant child is of my grandmother Remedios, or what I called her, Nanay, smiling and eating while engaging in loud conversation with the numerous other Filipino migrant caregivers who shared our table in the '90s. Remedios was an excellent cook—*menudo* and *pecadillo* were some of the dishes that would draw crowds on a Sunday. As a nine-year-old child, I remember hanging out around the dinner table even after I'd had my fill, to listen—listen to the jokes, or the sad stories, or the memories of the provinces, or what was happening in the Philippines, whether crisis or celebration. I liked seeing how the plates full of rice, *ulam* (an entrée), and *patis* (fish sauce) would slowly empty while the voices of the family and community members would grow. As I collected the Corelle plates and the utensils, the lulls in laughter would turn into serious conversation—my cue to go to the garage and play with the other kids. Over the kitchen table, over steamed rice desserts and hot water, the Filipino migrants in my life would exchange essential information about filing for "amnesty," a possible legalization route for undocumented migrants; which immigration lawyers were to be trusted and which weren't; who knew of new jobs; who was cycling through a horrible employer; which family needed the pot in the monthly giving circle; whose family member was ailing. The rich conversation, the *kuwentuhan*, among migrant workers over food and laughter was at once a community-building social process and an exchange of essential information among peers, especially for the newcomer immigrants working in the caregiving industry.

As a scholar and activist, I have never wandered too far from the essential chatter of the kitchen table among Filipino immigrants. It has and will always be a homeplace for me; the sounds, smells, and practice teach me that care and care work show up in the most mundane of spaces. Food is a staple in any Filipino migrant worker organizing event or gathering. While many of the caregivers I've worked and organized with over the years are not wealthy financially, they have repeatedly been able to eke out a few dollars to bring a dish or snack to our gatherings—an offering of sorts. They offer their humble contributions of a savory Filipino dish or a sweet treat as a way to commune. Before I had my children, I reveled at the generosity of care workers when they brought their regional dishes like fish *lumpia*, oxtail *kare-kare*, or *adobong puti* to the table of kuwentuhan. Before a word was even spoken, I was invited to a table to be part of a community. As the mother of two beautiful children, Aya Gabriela and Cy Andres, I understand the inclination to start with food—with them there's always a request for a snack or a question about when we will be eating next. When I have my children in tow to protests and organizing meetings, food signals that there is communing to be held rather than a mere transaction. Instinctively, they approach a food table at a community event, gather some items, and find a comfy seat.

This painstakingly careful and longitudinal table I have painted is my attempt at drawing a through line across time and geography as to what it can look like to care for caregivers, an idea that is simple on the surface yet complex below. To honor the lives and work of caregivers, it is essential that we value their dignity, respect their humanity, and attend to their basic needs. While the political and economic conditions in the United States are constantly in flux, the contradictions in the work and lives of care workers has yet to spark the social imagination of Americans, even if communities have steadily organized local and national campaigns, developed organizations and policy, and created multimedia efforts to illuminate the history of organizing domestic workers.[1] There is still a need to enjoin people in the thousands to take part in building migrant worker power, to remind people that there is a seat for everyone at this table. One of the questions we can grapple with is the scale of the essential nature of care work and the migrant workers who do this work.

The COVID-19 pandemic changed everything, for everyone. In fact, on a global scale, the lives of Filipina/o migrant workers all over the world were upended. Much of their livelihood was interrupted by the pandemic. In the weeks after shelter-in-place mandates spread from country to country, overseas Filipino workers were repatriated en masse from their posts on land and sea.[2] Panicked and unprepared, the Philippine state responded poorly to the massive return migration as they struggled to deal with the pandemic within the country's borders.[3] The labor export–oriented institutions designed for outmigration in the Philippines collapsed under the weight of the sheer numbers of overseas Filipino workers who needed to be repatriated.[4]

Scholars and nongovernmental organizations have argued that multiple and multilevel problems arose as thousands of land- and sea-based workers were repatriated.[5] Coordination among emaciated social-serving governmental departments such as the Department of Public Health, Bureau of Quarantine, and Department of Tourism (for hotel accommodations, etc.), and the multiple migration-related agencies such as the Philippine Overseas Employment Agency and the Overseas Workers Welfare Agency were convoluted. Protocols of testing, duration of quarantine, food and drink, and the process of receiving repatriated workers differed from region to region, resulting in "locally stranded individuals" at port cities like Manila and Cebu City.[6] At the height of lockdown and return migration, regions of the Philippines were closing and not receiving overseas Filipino workers, who carried a social stigma as carriers of the COVID-19 virus. Under, then-president Rodrigo Roa Duterte's administration, the government employed a "wait and see" approach in response to the global health pandemic. And when the virus began to spread in the country, the administration rolled out the strictest and most militarized efforts to institute "community quarantines" nationwide.[7] The Philippine state's ineffective policies to manage the pandemic, and, arguably, the ongoing pandemic, stems from its neoliberal servitude and dependence on export-oriented, global capitalist countries like the United States and China. While labor brokerage and the export of Filipinos has been the Philippines' saving grace in terms of geopolitical economics, COVID-19 proved that relying on migrant citizens to float any economy is a threadbare strategy that is sure to fail under crisis.

Migrants who were not forced to return to the Philippines experienced instability under expiring immigration or labor visas, social stigma pegging them as carriers of the virus, intensified workloads in industries deemed "essential"—in short, an exacerbation of the existing inequalities migrant workers face across the globe.[8] Migrant workers who were not repatriated, such as domestic workers in Hong Kong and Canada or seafarers in oil tankers at sea, experienced increased mental health stressors as their work conditions became nonstop because of lockdown and immobility mandates.[9] On the other hand, people working in hospitality and tourism or construction were stranded and laid off by the companies and agencies that hired them but could not keep workers employed. These overseas Filipino workers were homeless and unable to remit funds to their families in the Philippines.[10] When stranded migrants were finally able to come home, their start-and-stop journeys from their diasporic location to their home communities extended the time away from their families and time without work and wages. Additionally, even if migrants engaged in continuous work abroad for many years, their daily living costs and regular remittances did not set up them or their families with savings.[11] With a shoddy plan for reintegration, the Philippine state did not and could not offer reasonable or sustainable jobs for return migrants. Through the lockdown period, and as pandemic conditions disallowed labor migration, aspiring migrants in the Philippines saw their plans for training, education, and eventual labor migration restricted and delayed.[12] To this day, as opportunities for short-term and long-term labor contracts return, Filipinos in the Philippines are weighing the gamble of labor migration while the collective memory of repatriation and immobility is still fresh.[13]

Caregivers described in this book, I argue, belong in the discussion of how COVID-19 affected overseas Filipino workers and migrant workers, more broadly, at a global scale. While some of them might not identify as an Overseas Filipino Worker or OFW, a Philippine state label denoting people employed with a temporary, short-term labor contract in regions like the Middle East or the Asia-Pacific, and perhaps would rather consider themselves emigrants to the United States without a perspective of returning to the Philippines, what they have in common with their counterparts in the Filipino labor diaspora are that they are migrant citizens who were working abroad during a global pandemic, sending money to their families in the Philippines as workers in precarious industries. In many ways, this global and transnational perspective is an essential viewpoint to understand the context and plight of Filipino caregivers in the States, especially in the time of coronavirus. Caregivers gritted their teeth through uncertain work conditions and accepted increased workloads through shelter-in-place restrictions, suffering from the invisibility of their positions as frontliners, surviving and contracting the virus as they attended to the most vulnerable populations. Without regard for worker health and safety, the health-care industry understood the significance of eldercare and long-term care facilities yet did not and could not advocate for proper staffing or effective enforcement of basic protections like personal protective equipment.[14] While it is unclear how many caregivers and health professionals in nonhospital settings died from COVID-19 as a result of their uninterrupted work in the pandemic, it is clear that the transnational obligations of migrant workers fastened them to unsafe working conditions.

As political economic institutions and states across the world collaborated (or not) in creating policies and regulations for migrant workers, it was clear that logics of racial capitalism were at work in dispersing and disposing of migrant workers when the axles of capital slowed to a halt. In what Katherine Nasol calls the "neoliberal governance of care," Filipino caregivers' experiences before and during the pandemic only brought to light the crises of the privatized US care industry.[15] The first and existing crisis, as I discussed in other parts of this book, is the emaciated eldercare and long-term care industry, which has become an afterthought in the American social and political narrative around health and aging.[16] Even if there is a certainty of an increase in demand for eldercare in the United States, there is no political will to properly examine and fund changes that might bring about equitable working conditions and standardizing pay and benefits for care workers.[17] Scholars have established that the working conditions and job stressors for Filipino immigrants, especially in precarious industries like caregiving and domestic work, have negative impacts on their health outcomes.[18] Even if there is ample evidence that Filipino caregivers' physical and mental health suffer under occupational stressors, the caregiving industry continues to capitalize on Filipinos' newcomer status and transnational obligations wherein their class positions are dangerously close to or living under the US poverty line. Given that domestic work in the country has a racialized and gendered history of exploiting care work and care workers, it is important to understand that Filipinos did not just haphazardly end up at the bottom rung of the US health-care system.[19] Rather, as scholars of racial capitalism teach us, Filipinos, as racialized laboring bodies, are assigned a particular value to maintain whiteness and wealth for profit and capital accumulation.[20]

The global COVID-19 pandemic was a crisis in and of itself, and it exposed the withered eldercare system in the United States as many settings of long-term care became hot spots of COVID-19 transmissions. While these sites were, in fact, front lines in the fight against COVID-19, care workers, nurses, and administrative staff bore the brunt of early onset of the virus as they adapted to new and ever-changing health conditions without the recognition and funding to properly protect care workers. Because the health-care and eldercare system buckled under the weight of an unprecedented global health crisis, the acute and long-term impacts on care workers' physical and mental health were not documented across the industry.[21] The many labor standards that were breached during the pandemic, such as low staffing, inadequate protective equipment, overtime pay, sick leave, and racial discrimination, have not been tracked across the industry and over time. In some ways, the dual crises of the eldercare industry and the COVID-19 pandemic continues. In the future, caregivers could use scholar-activists as allies in creating validated measures and surveys that can assist in tracking the mental and physical health outcomes of home health-care workers. There is a need to create tools to track the types of labor rights infringement that are unrestrained in the current model of long-term care.

Despite these conditions, caregivers across the many phases of my research reminded me of the abundance of care among them. Their care for their own transnational families and their willingness to expand their communality of caring among them were not restricted by the labor and political systems bereft of care governing their daily work. Under the COVID-19 pandemic, caregivers at workplaces readily took up shifts when coworkers fell ill and shared the information they received through word-of-mouth or text messages. They built a network among themselves and their family members to deliver cooked food and groceries to ailing coworkers. Away from the families in the Philippines, many caregivers on invisible front lines continued to communicate through the virtual channels they'd been operating on for decades.[22] Across the Filipino labor diaspora, they communicated with family members working in domestic work or health care in various countries all over the world serving on COVID front lines. While they were carved out of information systems in the American health-care industry, they became creative in obtaining facts about the virus and how to protect themselves. Organizations like PAWIS in San Jose organized delivery drop-offs of personal protective equipment such as gloves and masks, even including homemade ginger teas called *salabat* and banana bread to the "care packages" they left on the porches of care homes. They recruited their children, nieces and nephews, and grandchildren to make deliveries, to help access COVID-19 tests and vaccine appointments. These practices were termed "mutual aid" in the pandemic, but for caregivers, this is how such supplies moved in the world before the pandemic hit. While the dual crisis of eldercare and COVID-19 wreaked havoc on the lives of caregivers, they demonstrated that their innovation and creativity would not be constrained. In fact, they drew from a well of relentless activism and service to one another as external conditions insisted on not only their social but also their political isolation.

CARING ACROSS FILIPINO GENERATIONS

Yet, Filipina/o caregivers in the San Francisco Bay Area did not live through the onset of the COVID-19 pandemic in a vacuum. While caregivers were invisible frontliners in the battle to slow the transmission of COVID, they were also living in multigenerational households with family members working as essential workers across health sectors as hospital administrators, nurses, medical staff, and public health workers.[23] Although Filipino Americans represent only 4 percent of nurses in the United States, their presence in intensive and acute care units during the pandemic put them at a particularly high risk for COVID-19 death. In fact, studies showed that over 30 percent of COVID-19 deaths in nurses in the States were from the Filipino American community.[24] While there is a lack of consistent and disaggregated data to analyze the mortality rates of Filipino Americans in health care, their overrepresentation across various sectors can be one way to explain these statistics. Across work sectors, Filipinos in the United States were affected gravely by the pandemic. In California, early in the pandemic over a third of deaths in Asian Americans due to COVID-19 were Filipino American, even if Filipino Americans comprised only 25 percent of the Asian American population in the state.[25] When we accept that Filipino migrant workers in the United States have and continue to be brought into the American racial and class order as exploitable and disposable workers, it is clear that their overrepresentation in health-care sectors correlates to COVID-19 deaths and is thus part of the necropolitical rubric that extends American imperialism across the Pacific to recruit migrant workers and back again to the States.[26]

For young Filipina/o Americans who shared these very same households in the San Francisco Bay Area with older siblings and kin who worked as caregivers, nurses, and in various health sectors, COVID proved to be a way to understand how a global pandemic reaches into intimate relationships, those of our kin and family members. The 1.5- and second-generation Filipina/o Americans with whom I've had the privilege of collaborating often intellectually understood the sacrifices that their elders and previous generations in their families made to help them achieve the futures they envisioned—for example, finishing up a baccalaureate degree or obtaining a stable job. During the pandemic it was clear that many of them developed a different view of these sacrifices. I was told anecdotal stories about how older sisters or mothers working as nurses and caregivers came home from a commute or their workplace, changing in their garages and laundering their clothes immediately upon setting foot in their homes. During kuwentuhan, young people reported that they did not spend quality time with their health-care worker family members for months as they quarantined in one area of the house to protect the rest of the family members, FaceTiming or text messaging as a way to stay in touch even under the same roof.

In a reflection paper shared by one of my research collaborators, Kristal, a 1.5-generation Filipinx immigrant who was in their early twenties when they started as a collaborator, wrote:

> An issue that one of the [workers] is currently facing reminded me of my own struggle which was regarding transportation. One of the [workers] does not have a car and has to travel 2 hours to their work. This reminded me how when my dad had COVID-19, he was the only one who can drive so I felt really guilty for not knowing how to drive to be able to help out my parents get to places, do errands for our household or even just for my mom and I to get tested for the virus. I feel like having a car and being able to drive is a privilege right now. However, some of them use Uber to get to places but sometimes choose not to or only use it after taking a bus when their destination is closer so that they can save money as Uber rides are quite expensive.

Kristal's acknowledgment of the parallels between their experience with commuting and traveling and their own parents exhibits how participating in kuwentuhan allowed them to reflect on the similar challenges faced by their family members. While circumstances were different between care workers in our study and their parents, Kristal found enough distance from their personal life to understand that the impacts of the pandemic on their own family were akin to other Filipino families struggling through basic needs such as transport.

Although Kristal's own immigrant trajectory, their academic training, and political activism on the SF State campus has shaped their continued involvement in progressive Filipino organizing in the Bay Area, I believe that their participation in the CARE Project and kuwentuhan became a touchpoint in building their political imagination and action. Kristal's acknowledgment of the issues care workers faced during the pandemic gave them pause to observe the commonalities between their parents' daily struggles and those of other migrants. To be able to step out of one's own experience and recognize a collective story is a powerful outcome of kuwentuhan as a method.[27] Kuwentuhan encourages a practice of weaving one's story with one another during the actual discussion and beyond. For Kristal, and many of my research collaborators who identified as 1.5- and second-generation immigrants, the woven fabric of kuwentuhan was a practice in extending a social and political imaginary toward involvement in Filipino American service and organizing. The trajectories of my research collaborators range from community organizers for issues like human rights in the Philippines and local Filipino migrant services, working in county-level mental health agencies focused on Asian Pacific Americans, and graduate programs in public health and educational psychology. While I don't claim that their paths all started from their work in CARE Project kuwentuhan sessions, I assert that their participation in kuwentuhan and research with Filipina/o care workers shaped their ideas on how social science research can be in service to our community. And for that, and for them, I am grateful.

For young people, the social isolation in the pandemic often produced increased levels of depression and anxiety that derailed some from achieving success in their academics and weakened their peer and familial relations.[28] While studies show that perseverance and grit became important psychological adaptations for Filipina/o Americans, it remains unclear how these social processes have come to be.[29] In this book, I have suggested that kuwentuhan and intergenerational dialogue can be one way that young people and elders in the Filipino community in the United States can reach some understanding with one another. In the past, I have suggested that kuwentuhan and participatory methodologies can be conscientizing processes for migrant workers.[30] And here I argue that intentional involvement and recruitment across age and immigrant generations can also engender similar processes of solidarity building, consciousness raising, and intergenerational activism.

I do not propose that kuwentuhan alone can spark and sustain activism. I do suggest that participatory methods and the democratization of social science methods, in a way that centers on building the political power and cultural practices of Filipinos, can be a generative tactic in creating opportunities for learning and dialogue across class backgrounds, work sectors, immigrant generations, and age cohorts in Filipino diasporic communities. Organizers, community members and leaders, students, and practitioners can consider the role of research and community-accountable researchers as a part of strategic planning in creating winnable campaigns, sustained political education, and building mass organizations.[31] Both the process, which can include kuwentuhan (or versions of it), and the types of data collected can be powerful methods of telling and sharing stories to build bridges of understanding and portals of belonging across immigrant generations and age cohorts. The multiple iterations of the CARE Project and continuing to conduct research in the early stages of the pandemic demonstrated the potential in exchange and connection as a catalyst for solidarity and garnering support to advocate for migrant workers' rights. Moving forward, I look forward to scholars and activists developing social science research methods that are rooted in culturally accountable and responsive ways partnered with community organizations to build a robust intergenerational community of activism and political engagement. As Filipinx scholars continue to draw from histories and contemporary movements of their culture's diasporic activism, there is a need for a Filipinx American methodology to emerge from collaboration and participation from scholars, students, activists, and community members.[32]

The power of kuwentuhan is in the practice of communal care it can offer to all of its participants. In the midst of the pandemic, for me as a mother of two young children, one a toddler and the other a preschooler, contending with the realities of a global pandemic while transitioning into virtual teaching and work from home, and for my partner, the shelter-in-place days became long and arduous. The virtual kuwentuhan via Zoom with Filipino care workers and Filipina/o American students became a salve for the social isolation we were all experiencing. Below is an excerpt from my field notes from a Zoom kuwentuhan in August 2020:

> I was feeling so tired today. Logging on to Zoom at 7pm, I felt like I wish I asked a research collaborator to head this up on their own instead of me. 7pm in my life right now feels like 11pm. Dinner time, bath time, bedtime and barely tip toeing out of the kids room as they drifted off to sleep, I was surprised I didn't fall asleep on their room floor. I didn't know how I was gonna get myself together to hold space for the kuwentuhan.
>
> But as soon as the caregivers started to trickle in, I found a boost of energy. Tita Tess introduced caregivers as each of them came into the Zoom room. Small talk ensued, laughter and giggling over inside jokes were traded. We would go loud then quiet for the first 20 minutes of our time together waiting for people to iron out their technical Zoom questions. While my students called workers to restart the app on their iPads or phones, I started with a check in question, "What have you eaten for dinner?" Many of them hadn't eaten yet, and didn't have plans to since they were at work or on the Zoom with me. And it donned [sic] on me, I hadn't eaten yet either. So before we started the formal kuwentuhan, all of us pushed each other to go get food or a drink and the check in was to show what we were going to eat as we talked.

Food and kuwentuhan go together; like a fried fish and a savory broth with rice for dinner. These field notes remind me that kuwentuhan was a space of care for me too. It was a time when I could share how hard it was for me to attend to the domestic work of my family, even with my husband, Raul, sharing the labor with me. Similar to and different from care workers and young people in the kuwentuhan session, we were all struggling with the labor of care as the world shut down.

Whether it was the absence of child-care providers, nannies, housekeepers, teachers or professors, restaurants, or caregivers, so many of us—and, arguably, across the country and the globe—could really feel the difference when workers who attended to social reproductive labor were all of a sudden gone. For the care workers on Zoom, their work continued at an intensified rate, while those of us who didn't work in their industry tried to patch together our lives without the essential work of paid domestic labor. During the time of the pandemic, it was so clear to me that domestic labor was some of the most important work in the world. Thus, kuwentuhan, before, during, and after the pandemic, also humanized all parts of me too. As we began the Zoom kuwentuhan with a spoonful of rice and soup or a granola bar or mango juice, the experience lifted me up as many of the workers, some of whom I had just met for the first time on Zoom, led with care in the question "Did you eat yet?"

HEALTH AND DIGNITY FOR CARE WORKERS

The California Domestic Workers Coalition (CDWC) has been and continues to be a powerful contemporary social movement that has inspired and guided my interventions as a scholar-activist in service of building migrant worker power. In 2013 the leadership of Filipina and Latina nannies, housekeepers, care workers, and other domestic workers in the CDWC, resulted in then-governor Jerry Brown's signing of the California Domestic Workers Bill of Rights (AB241-Ammiano). The mass organizations across California persevered over a six-year legislative campaign that included two vetoes to clinch the victory of the bill of rights. While the final version of the law was modest compared to the original demands of the coalition, it extended overtime protections to personal attendants (such as nannies and home-care attendants) with the condition that the law would expire in three years. In 2016 the CDWC made the provisions of AB241 permanent under SB1015 (Leyva). More important, the legislative campaign worked with innovative organizing tactics to build worker leadership in migrant organizations up and down California, especially with immigrant women of color across race, ethnicity, and language.

The coalition pulled in multiple stakeholders such as Hand in Hand Domestic Employers Network, professors and students from universities, legal partners and law centers, and many more.³³ In 2018 and 2019 the CDWC focused its advocacy efforts on securing funds to create an education and outreach program, housed within the California Division of Labor Standards Enforcement (DLSE), geared toward increasing the awareness of and compliance with the provisions of the bill of rights. In 2019 funds were allocated to support the first-of-its-kind education program within the DLSE that would rely on partnerships with community organizations to inform both employers and domestic workers about existing labor protections. During the pandemic and in the years that followed, the CDWC utilized, and continues to engage in, virtual, hybrid, and in-person actions to advance campaigns to protect the health and dignity of domestic workers. Following a veto in 2020, the coalition won SB321 in 2021 to create an advisory board that ultimately wrote the first-ever industry-specific guidelines for health and safety for domestic workers and day laborers adopted through Cal/OSHA (California Occupational Safety and Health Act) in December 2022.³⁴ Currently, worker leaders in the coalition are leading a legislative campaign to pass SB686 (Durazo) to establish health and safety as a right for domestic workers and to continue to expand education and outreach to employers, educating and supporting them to adapt the aforementioned guidelines and recommendations.

I end with the work of the coalition because just as much as the political influence of the eldercare industry toward for-profit models of eldercare and long-term care is apparent in shaping the lives of Filipino care workers, it is abundantly clear that the political power and organizing of migrant workers, especially immigrant women of color, must be held as a model of radical care and hope. In my involvement with the CDWC, I have sat through meetings, political education discussions, milestone celebrations, and capitol mobilizations where translation and interpretation are non-negotiable; where child care is a staple given that many workers and worker leaders raise their own families while they participate in political work; where food and drink are a certainty because community members often attend these events after work; where a politics of care requires that coalition leaders pay close attention to how we relate to one another while building oppositional power to the status quo. These examples of interpretation, child care, and food and drink are attuned to the kitchen table chatter that came so naturally to my grandmother and her colleagues in the early 1990s. They are examples of recognizing one another's whole selves and making room for them at the table, or at the meeting, or at the event, or at the rally. Many of these intentional practices come from acknowledging that, first and foremost, we are human beings in relation with one another. And we must care for one another—that doing so might be an important part of building communities of care, and mass organizations, mass movements, community centers, statewide coalitions and, frankly, our daily relationships. Dear reader, it is my privilege to be able to share with you these moments of radical care and solidarity, and I ask you to think about how *you* think, create, and act with this perspective—to make care an essential part of your politic. Not only because it has shaped mine but also because it might be the key to revaluing care in our daily lives and, hopefully, one day on a systems scale.

In this book my hope has been to provide a sustained look at the lives and collective plight of Filipina/o caregivers. I wrote about their day-to-day working conditions and the normalization of their exploitation in the long-term care industry, especially during the COVID-19 pandemic. My aim has been to offer the basis for why they, and why we, should all be figuring out how we can join and support the local, state-level, and national campaigns to secure the health, safety, and dignity of domestic workers. It has been my privilege to share how care workers taught me what communities of care can look, taste, and feel like and, necessarily, how their care work, both paid and unpaid, will affect generations after them. I hope that writing about the potential of intergenerational care in both research and activism can be a way forward to activate dialogue and, eventually, solidarity and political organizing. I leave you with these examples of radical care among communities, across generations, political organizations, research projects, and coalition building because, truly, my hope is that you will join us.

NOTES

INTRODUCTION

1. Cranford, *Home Care Fault Lines*; Nazareno, Parreñas, and Fan, "Can I Ever Retire?"

2. Roberts, "Psychosocial Effects of Workplace Hazardous Exposures."

3. Dilworth-Anderson, Williams, and Cooper, "The Contexts of Experiencing Emotional Distress among Family Caregivers to Elderly African Americans."

4. Clergé, *The New Noir*; Robinson, *Black Marxism*.

5. Day, *Alien Capital*.

6. Gonzalves and Labrador, *Filipinos in Hawaiʻi*; Mabalon, *Little Manila Is in the Heart*; Choy, *Empire of Care*.

7. Chang, *Disposable Domestics*.

8. Nasol, "The Governance of Care."

9. Boris and Klein, *Caring for America*.

10. Tung, "The Cost of Caring."

11. Brennan et al., "The Marketisation of Care"; Macdonald and Charlesworth, "Cash for Care under the NDIS."

12. Armstrong and Armstrong, *The Privatization of Care*.

13. Harrington, Pollock, and Sutaria, "Privatization of Nursing Homes in the United Kingdom and the United States."

14. Geraci, Hutchison, and Brunt, "California's Newly Reformed Residential Care Facilities for the Elderly."

15. Riley, Nazareno, and Malish, "24-Hour Care."

16. Shah, "Understaffed and Overworked."

17. Nadasen, *Care*.

18. Iecovich, "What Makes Migrant Live-In Home Care Workers in Elder Care

Be Satisfied with Their Job?"; Chowdhury and Gutman, "Migrant Live-In Caregivers Providing Care to Canadian Older Adults."

19. Ayalon, "Family and Family-Like Interactions in Households with Round-the-Clock Paid Foreign Carers in Israel"; Faul et al., "Promoting Sustainability In Frontline Home Care Aides."

20. Todd, *Valley of Heart's Delight*; Tsu, *Garden of the World*.

21. Tsu, *Garden of the World*.

22. Nasol, "The Governance of Care."

23. Hossfeld, "Hiring Immigrant Women"; Pellow and Park, *The Silicon Valley of Dreams*; Pitti, *The Devil in Silicon Valley*.

24. Pellow and Park, *The Silicon Valley of Dreams*.

25. Smith and Woodward, *The Legacy of High Tech Development*.

26. Vergara, *Pinoy Capital*.

27. Tabb, *The Amoral Elephant*.

28. Bonus, *Locating Filipino Americans*; Vergara, *Pinoy Capital*.

29. Occupational Safety and Health Administration, "Guidelines for Nursing Homes."

30. Geraci, Hutchison, and Brunt, "California's Newly Reformed Residential Care Facilities for the Elderly."

31. Shah, "Understaffed and Overworked."

32. Riley, Nazareno, and Malish, "24-Hour Care."

33. Browne, Braun, and Arnsberger, "Filipinas as Residential Long-Term Care Providers"; Nazareno, "Welfare State Replacements."

34. Francisco-Menchavez, Celemen, and Osorio, "Filipino Formal Caregivers to the Elderly and Normalized Exploitation in the Workplace."

35. Rodriguez, *Migrants for Export*; Guevarra, *Marketing Dreams, Manufacturing Heroes*.

36. Huang, Yeoh, and Toyota, "Caring for the Elderly."

37. Ortiga and Macabasag, "Temporality and Acquiescent Immobility among Aspiring Nurse Migrants in the Philippines"; Ortiga and Macabasag, "Understanding International Immobility through Internal Migration."

38. Baas and Yeoh, "Introduction."

39. Choy, *Empire of Care*.

40. Yeoh and Huang, "'Home' and 'Away.'"

41. Guevarra, *Marketing Dreams, Manufacturing Heroes*; Rodriguez, *Migrants for Export*.

42. Gilmore discusses this dynamic and politics of abolition. See Gilmore, *Abolition Geography*.

43. Glenn, "From Servitude to Service Work."

44. Cranford and Chun, "Multi-level Analyses of Homecare Labor," 387.

45. Fraser, "Capitalism's Crisis of Care."

46. Osterman, *Who Will Care for Us?*

47. Bezanson and Luxton, *Social Reproduction*; Bhattacharya, *Social Reproduction Theory*; Federici, "Social Reproduction Theory."

48. Federici, *Wages against Housework*; Beneria, "The Enduring Debate over Unpaid Labour"; Dalla Costa, "Capitalism and Reproduction."

49. Laslett and Brenner, "Gender and Social Reproduction."

50. Bezanson and Luxton, *Social Reproduction*; Bhattacharya, *Social Reproduction Theory*; Federici, "Social Reproduction Theory."

51. Colen, "Stratified Reproduction and West Indian Childcare Workers and Employers in New York."

52. Davis, *Women, Race & Class*.

53. Nishida, *Just Care*.

54. Navarro, "The Labor Process and Health."

55. Hossfeld, "Hiring Immigrant Women"; Roberts, "Psychosocial Effects of Workplace Hazardous Exposures"; Smith and Woodward, *The Legacy of High Tech Development*.

56. Nasol and Francisco-Menchavez, "Filipino Home Care Workers."

57. Cranford, *Home Care Fault Lines*.

58. Nasol, "The Governance of Care."

59. Francisco, "From Where I Sit"; Jocson, "Whose Story Is It Anyway?"

60. Gordon et al., "Balancing Caregiving and Work"; Pilkonis et al., "Item Banks for Measuring Emotional Distress from the Patient-Reported Outcomes Measurement Information System (PROMIS®)."

61. Francisco-Menchavez, Celemen, and Osorio, "Filipino Formal Caregivers to the Elderly and Normalized Exploitation in the Workplace."

CHAPTER 1 / NO WORK, NO PAY

1. Tung, "The Cost of Caring."

2. Williams and Dilworth-Anderson, "Systems of Social Support in Families Who Care for Dependent African American Elders."

3. Cranford, *Home Care Fault Lines*; Glenn, "Racial Ethnic Women's Labor."

4. Guevarra, "The Balikbayan Researcher."

5. Duffy, "Doing the Dirty Work"; Glenn, "From Servitude to Service Work"; Nadasen, *Household Workers Unite*.

6. Bhattacharya, *Social Reproduction Theory*.

7. Laslett and Brenner, "Gender and Social Reproduction," 383.

8. Boris and Klein, "Frontline Caregivers."

9. Nadasen, "Citizenship Rights, Domestic Work, and the Fair Labor Standards Act."

10. Asis, Huaang, and Yeoh, "When the Light of the Home Is Abroad"; Bryceson and Vuorela, *The Transnational Family*; Espiritu, *Home Bound*; Francisco-Menchavez, *The Labor of Care*; Guevarra, *Marketing Dreams, Manufacturing Heroes*; Yeoh, Willis, and Fakhri, "Introduction."

11. Nadasen, "Citizenship Rights, Domestic Work, and the Fair Labor Standards Act."

12. Braedley et al., "We're Told, 'Suck It Up.'"

13. Dutta, "Health Meanings among Foreign Domestic Workers in Singapore."

14. Watson, *Sociology, Work and Industry*; Cranford, *Home Care Fault Lines*; Chang, *Disposable Domestics*; Nazareno, "Welfare State Replacements."

15. Boris and Klein, "Frontline Caregivers."

16. Nazareno, Parreñas, and Fan, "Can I Ever Retire?"

17. Francisco-Menchavez, "Filipino Formal Caregivers to the Elderly and Normalized Exploitation in the Workplace."

18. Nazareno, Parreñas, and Fan, "Can I Ever Retire?"; Shah, "Understaffed and Overworked."

19. Nasol and Francisco-Menchavez, "Filipino Home Care Workers."

20. David, *Brown Skin, White Minds*; Tamanal, Park, and Kim, "The Relationship of Perceived Stress and Lifestyle Choices among Filipino Adolescents."

21. David, *Brown Skin, White Minds*.

CHAPTER 2 / INVISIBLE FRONTLINERS IN THE TIME OF CORONAVIRUS

1. Attal, Lurie, and Neumark, "A Rapid Assessment of Migrant Careworkers' Psychosocial Status during Israel's COVID-19 Lockdown"; Bismark et al., *Experiences of Health Workers in the COVID-19 Pandemic*.

2. Reid, Ronda-Perez, and Schenker, "Migrant Workers, Essential Work, and COVID-19."

3. Giordano, "Freedom or Money?"

4. Tessler, Choi, and Kao, "The Anxiety of Being Asian American," 636–646; Jeung and Nham, "Incidents of Coronavirus-Related Discrimination."

5. Bismark et al., *Experiences of Health Workers in the COVID-19 Pandemic*.

6. Vizheh et al., "The Mental Health of Healthcare Workers in the COVID-19 Pandemic."

7. Banta and Pratt, *Immobilised by the Pandemic*, 557.

8. Bismark et al., *Experiences of Health Workers in the COVID-19 Pandemic*.

9. Nadasen, "Citizenship Rights, Domestic Work, and the Fair Labor Standards Act."

10. Siu and Chun, "Yellow Peril and Techno-Orientalism in the Time of Covid-19," 421–440.

11. M. Kang, *The Managed Hand*.

12. Li and Galea, "Racism and the COVID-19 Epidemic."

13. de Borja, "Overseas Filipino Workers and the COVID-19 Pandemic."

14. Cabalquinto, "Ambivalent Intimacies"; Cabalquinto, "'We're Not Only Here but We're There in Spirit"; Francisco, "The Internet Is Magic"; Uy-Tioco and Cabalquinto, "Transnational Mobile Carework."

15. Thompson, "The Philippines' Business Process Outsourcing Industry through COVID-19."

16. Asis, "Repatriating Filipino Migrant Workers in the Time of the Pandemic"; Fernandez et al., "A Hero's Welcome?"; Ortiga and Macabasag, "Understanding International Immobility through Internal Migration."

17. Francisco-Menchavez, *The Labor of Care*.

18. Perrea, "The Echoes of Slavery."

19. Nadasen, *Household Workers Unite*; Verret, "How Racist Policies Continue to Hurt Home Care Workers."

20. Shah, "Understaffed and Overworked."

21. Shah, "Understaffed and Overworked."

22. Delgado, "The Health Impacts of Domestic Labor on Women Workers in Massachusetts."

23. Braedley et al., "We're Told, 'Suck It Up.'"

24. Delgado, "The Health Impacts of Domestic Labor on Women Workers in Massachusetts."

CHAPTER 3 / RELATIONALITY AS A POLITICS OF CARE

1. Nasol and Francisco-Menchavez, "Filipino Home Care Workers."

2. Laslett and Brenner, "Gender and Social Reproduction"; Bezanson and Luxton, *Social Reproduction*.

3. Kofman, "Rethinking Care through Social Reproduction"; Tungohan, "Reconceptualizing Motherhood, Reconceptualizing Resistance."

4. Bhattacharya, *Social Reproduction Theory*.

5. de Borja, "Overseas Filipino Workers and the COVID-19 Pandemic."

6. Tadiar, *Fantasy Production*.

7. Tadiar, *Fantasy Production*, 244.

8. Isaac, *Filipino Time*.

9. Isaac, *Filipino Time*, 16.

10. Nasol and Francisco-Menchavez, "Filipino Home Care Workers"; Nazareno, "Welfare State Replacements"; Tung, "The Cost of Caring."

11. Hobart and Kneese, "Radical Care," 1.

12. Tronto, "Creating Caring Institutions."

13. Cranford, *Home Care Fault Lines*.

14. Folbre, *The Invisible Heart*.

15. Isaac, *Filipino Time*.

16. England, "Emerging Theories of Care Work"; Hochschild, *The Managed Heart*.

17. Francisco-Menchavez, Celemen, and Osorio, "Filipino Formal Caregivers to the Elderly and Normalized Exploitation in the Workplace."

18. Nazareno, "Welfare State Replacements."

19. Sabon, "Force, Fraud, and Coercion—What Do They Mean?" 457.

20. Chin and Villazor, *The Immigration and Nationality Act of 1965*; Francisco and Rodriguez, "Coming to America."

21. Eidelson, "Nurses Who Faced Lawsuits for Quitting Are Fighting Back"; McCarthy, "In Depth."

22. Fukushima, *Migrant Crossings*.

23. Fukushima, "An American Haunting."

24. Enriquez, *From Colonial to Liberation Psychology*.

25. David et al., "Losing Kapwa."

26. Alvarez and Juang, "Filipino Americans and Racism."

27. Nasol, "The Governance of Care."

28. Kang, *The Managed Hand*; Lowe, *Immigrant Acts*.

29. Francisco-Menchavez, *The Labor of Care*.

30. de Leon, "Pagod, Dugot, Pawis (Exhaustion, Blood, and Sweat)"; Tungohan, "Reconceptualizing Motherhood, Reconceptualizing Resistance."

31. Tadiar, *Fantasy Production*.

32. Nasol and Francisco-Menchavez, "Filipino Home Care Workers."

33. de Borja, "Overseas Filipino Workers and the COVID-19 Pandemic."

34. Woodly et al., "The Politics of Care," 1.

35. Tronto, "Creating Caring Institutions."

36. Nishida, *Just Care*.

37. Vilog and Piocos, "Community of Care amid Pandemic Inequality"; Woodly et al., "The Politics of Care"; Tungohan, *Care Activism*; Nasol, "The Governance of Care."

38. Colen, "Stratified Reproduction and West Indian Childcare Workers and Employers in New York."

39. Rodriguez, *Migrants for Export*; Guevarra, *Marketing Dreams, Manufacturing Heroes*.

40. Isaac, *Filipino Time*, 12.
41. Isaac, *Filipino Time*, 16.

CHAPTER 4 / KUWENTUHAN AND INTERGENERATIONAL ACTIVISM

1. Francisco-Menchavez et al., "Claiming Kapwa."
2. Atienza, "The Promise of Intimacy"; Espiritu, "Transnationalism and Filipino American Historiography"; Maramba and Museus, "The Utility of Using Mixed-Methods and Intersectionality Approaches"; Reyes, "Ethnographic Toolkit."
3. Piepzna-Samarasinha, *Care Work*.
4. Guevarra, *Marketing Dreams, Manufacturing Heroes*; Tyner, *The Philippines*.
5. Rodriguez, *Migrants for Export*.
6. Mabalon, *Little Manila Is in the Heart*.
7. Lindio-McGovern and Wallimann, *Globalization and Third World Women*; Padios, *A Nation on the Line*.
8. Choy, *Empire of Care*; Ruiz, "Made for Export"; Paligutan, *Lured by the American Dream*; Parreñas, "The Gender Paradox in the Transnational Families of Filipino Migrant Women."
9. Alba, "Cohorts and the Dynamics of Ethnic Change," 213.
10. Rumbaut, "Ages, Life Stages, and Generational Cohorts."
11. Caballero et al., "'It's the Filipino Way.'"
12. Gutierrez, "A Family Affair"; Kares, "Practicing 'Enlightened Capitalism'"; Pido, *Migrant Returns*.
13. Enriquez, *From Colonial to Liberation Psychology*.
14. Francisco, "'The Internet Is Magic'"; Francisco-Menchavez, *The Labor of Care*; Francisco-Menchavez, "Kuwentuhan as a Method."
15. Cammarota and Fine, *Revolutionizing Education*; Fine and Torre, "Intimate Details"; Dill et al., "Oh, We Got Beef?!"; Guishard et al., "Toward Epistemological Ethics"; Guishard et al., "What We Not Finna Do"; Billies et al., "Participatory Action Research"; Krueger-Henney, "What Are We Listening For?"; Krueger-Henney, "Through Space into the Flesh"; Krueger-Henney and Ruglis, "PAR Is a Way of Life."
16. Guishard, "The False Paths, the Endless Labors, the Turns Now This Way and Now That"; Bautista, Martinez, and O'Brien, "The Youth Will Speak"; Tintiangco-Cubales et al., "Toward an Ethnic Studies Pedagogy"; Cammarota and Fine, *Revolutionizing Education*; Krueger-Henney, "Through Space into the Flesh"; Torre and Fine, "Participatory Action Research (PAR) by Youth"; Fields, *Risky Lessons*; Fine and Torre, "Intimate Details."
17. IBON Foundation, *IBON Manual on Facilitating Participatory Research*, 38.
18. Choudhry et al., "Health Promotion and Participatory Action Research with

South Asian Women"; Cristancho et al., "Listening to Rural Hispanic Immigrants in the Midwest"; Meyer et al., "Immigrant Women Implementing Participatory Research in Health Promotion"; Patel, Rajpathak, and Karasz, "Bangladeshi Immigrants in New York City"; Unger, "Participatory Health Research with Immigrant Communities in Germany."

19. van der Velde, Williamson, and Ogilvie, "Participatory Action Research"; Parrado, McQuiston, and Flippen, "Participatory Survey Research."

20. Minkler et al., "Using Community-Based Participatory Research to Design and Initiate a Study on Immigrant Worker Health and Safety in San Francisco's Chinatown Restaurants."

21. Mata-Codesal, Kloetzer, and Maiztegui-Oñate, "Strengths, Risks and Limits of Doing Participatory Research in Migration Studies."

22. Montero-Sieburth, "Who Gives 'Voice' or 'Empowers Migrants' in Participatory Action Research?"

23. Billies et al., "Participatory Action Research"; Francisco, "From Where I Sit"; Francisco, "'The Internet Is Magic'"; Francisco, "Migrante, Abante"; Francisco-Menchavez, "Kuwentuhan as a Method"; Francisco-Menchavez et al., "Filipino Formal Caregivers to the Elderly and Normalized Exploitation in the Workplace"; Francisco-Menchavez and Tungohan, "Mula sa masa, tungo sa masa, From the People, to the People."

24. Brabeck, Lykes, and Hershberg, "Framing Immigration to and Deportation from the United States"; Madriz, "Using Focus Groups with Lower Socioeconomic Status Latina Women."

25. Sanchez, "Let the People Speak."

26. Kahakalau, "Indigenous Heuristic Action Research"; L. Smith, *Decolonizing Methodologies*; Tuck, "Re-Visioning Action."

27. Orteza, *Pakikipagkuwentuhan*; Pe-Pua, "From Decolonizing Psychology to the Development of a Cross-Indigenous Perspective in Methodology."

28. Francisco-Menchavez and Carlos, "Kuwentuhan across Generations."

29. Shah, "Understaffed and Overworked."

30. Francisco, "'Ang Ating Iisang Kuwento': Our Collective Story."

31. Dutta et al., "Health Meanings among Foreign Domestic Workers in Singapore."

32. Francisco-Menchavez, "Kuwentuhan as a Method."

33. Francisco-Menchavez, "Kuwentuhan as a Method."

34. Francisco-Menchavez and Tungohan, "Mula sa masa, tungo sa masa, From the People, to the People."

35. Francisco-Menchavez et al., "Filipino Formal Caregivers to the Elderly and Normalized Exploitation in the Workplace."

36. See Yoo and Kim, *Caring across Generations*.

37. De Tona, Frisina, and Ganga, "Editorial."

38. Mata-Codesal et al., "Strengths, Risks, and Limits of Doing Participatory Research in Migration Studies."

39. Francisco, "'Ang Ating Iisang Kuwento': Our Collective Story."

40. Collie et al., "You Can't Clap with One Hand"; del Vecchio, Toomey, and Tuck, "Placing Photovoice."

41. Gutierrez, "Mediated Remittances."

42. Gutierrez, "A Family Affair," 229.

43. Soehl and Waldinger, "Inheriting the Homeland?"

44. Gutierrez, "Being Filipino without the Philippines"; Levitt and Waters, *The Changing Face of Home*.

45. Gutierrez, "Being Filipino without the Philippines."

46. Gutierrez, "A Family Affair."

47. Espiritu, *Home Bound*.

48. Bonus and Tiongson, *Filipinx American Studies*; Buenavista, Jayakumar, and Misa, "Contextualizing Asian American Education through Critical Race Theory."

49. Portes and Zhou, "The New Second Generation."

50. Ferrera, "The Transformative Impact of Cultural Portals on the Ethnic Identity Development of Second-Generation Filipino-American Emerging Adults"; Kodama and Laylo, "The Unique Context of Identity-Based Student Organizations in Developing Leadership."

51. Gutierrez, "Being Filipino without the Philippines."

52. Baldock, "Migrants and Their Parents."

53. Attias-Donfut and Cook, "Intergenerational Relationships in Migrant Families."

54. Francisco, "The Internet Is Magic"; Francisco-Menchavez, "Kuwentuhan as a Method."

55. Pe-Pua, "From Decolonizing Psychology to the Development of a Cross-Indigenous Perspective in Methodology."

56. de Leon and Pahinga Collective, "A Call to Rest"; Perillo, *Choreographing in Color*; Villegas, *Manifest Technique*; Tiongson, "On Rethinking the Politics and Possibilities of Joy"; Burns, "Masagana 99"; Castaneda and Jopanda, "Transpacific Freedom Dreams"; Critical Filipino Studies Collective, "Anti–Martial Law Syllabus"; Diaz, *Postcolonial Configurations*; Ong, "Care as Collective Revolution"; Sales, "#NeverAgainToMartialLaw"; Sales, "Martial Law Histories from a Critical Filipina/x/o American Perspective"; Sanchez, "Let the People Speak"; Schulze-Oechtering, "'Anti-Marcos Filipinos' and Other Anti-Imperialist Diasporas"; Amorao, Custodio-Tan, and Soriano, *Closer to Liberation*; Curammeng and Tintiangco-Cubales, "Growing Our Own Hope"; A. Daus-Magbual, R. Daus-Magbual, and Tintiangco-Cubales, "Pin@ y Educational PARtnerships"; Tintiangco-Cubales and Sacramento, "Practicing Pinayist Pedagogy";

Colting-Stol, "How Mutual Aid and Community Care Ignite Further Grassroots Organizing Possibilities for Long-Term Change"; Viola, "Toward a Filipino/a Critical (FilCrit) Pedagogy"; Rodriguez, *Filipino American Transnational Activism*.

57. Cahill, "'Why Do They Hate Us?'" 154.

58. Francisco-Menchavez, *The Labor of Care*.

59. Gutierrez, Piñon, and Valmocena, "Co-Creating Knowledge with Undocumented Filipino Students"; Jopanda, "Talk Story Methodologies (Kuwentuhan) Kuwentuhan."

EPILOGUE

1. Coll et al., "It's a Matter of Trust"; Guglielmo and Joffroy, "A History of Domestic Work and Worker Organizing."

2. Asis, "Repatriating Filipino Migrant Workers in the Time of the Pandemic"; Ortiga and Liao, "When a Pandemic Disrupts the Export of People."

3. Kang and Latoja, "COVID-19 and Overseas Filipino Workers."

4. Lan, "Shifting Borders and Migrant Workers' Im/Mobility"; Ortiga and Liao, "When a Pandemic Disrupts the Export of People."

5. Asis, "Repatriating Filipino Migrant Workers in the Time of the Pandemic"; Espia et al., "Into the Unknown"; International Organization for Migration, "COVID-19 Impact Assessment on Returned Overseas Filipino Workers."

6. Suzuki, "The Philippines' Response to COVID-19."

7. Teehankee, "Duterte's Pandemic Populism."

8. Oliva-Arocas et al., "Health of International Migrant Workers during the COVID-19 Pandemic."

9. Banta and Pratt, "Immobilised by the Pandemic"; Yeung et al., "Feeling Anxious amid the COVID-19 Pandemic."

10. Francisco-Menchavez, "Accumulating Delay"; Ullah, Nawaz, and Chattoraj, "Locked Up under Lockdown."

11. Saguin, "Returning Broke and Broken?"

12. Galam, "Futures on Hold."

13. Francisco-Menchavez, "Accumulating Delay"; Ortiga and Macabasag, "Temporality and Acquiescent Immobility among Aspiring Nurse Migrants in the Philippines."

14. Harrington and Jacobsen, "Nurse Staffing in Nursing Homes in Industrialized Countries."

15. Nasol, "The Governance of Care."

16. Boris and Klein, "Frontline Caregivers."

17. Armstrong et al., "The Crisis in the Nursing Home Labour Force."

18. De Castro, Gee, and Takeuchi, "Job-Related Stress and Chronic Health Con-

ditions among Filipino Immigrants"; De Castro, Gee, and Takeuchi, "Workplace Discrimination and Health among Filipinos in the United States."

19. Nadasen, *Household Workers Unite*.

20. Robinson, *Black Marxism*; Gilmore, "Fatal Couplings of Power and Difference."

21. Nasol and Francisco-Menchavez, "Filipino Home Care Workers."

22. Cabalquinto, *(Im)mobile Homes*.

23. Nasol and Francisco-Menchavez, "Filipino Home Care Workers"; Sangalang, "'I'm Sick of Being Called a Hero.'"

24. Escobedo, Morey, and Ponce, "Lost on the Frontline, and Lost in the Data."

25. Wong, "Little Noticed, Filipino Americans Are Dying of COVID-19 at an Alarming Rate."

26. Balce, *Body Parts of Empire*.

27. Pe-Pua, "From Decolonizing Psychology to the Development of a Cross-Indigenous Perspective in Methodology."

28. Litam and Oh, "Coping Strategies as Moderators of COVID-19 Racial Discrimination in Filipino Americans."

29. Datu and Fincham, "The Relational and Mental Health Payoffs of Staying Gritty during the COVID-19 Pandemic."

30. Francisco-Menchavez, "Kuwentuhan as a Method"; Francisco-Menchavez and Tungohan, "Mula sa masa, tungo sa masa, From the People, to the People."

31. Mitchell and Coll, "Ethnic Studies as a Site for Political Education."

32. Tungohan, *Care Activism*; Rodriguez, *Filipino American Transnational Activism*; Amorao, Custodio-Tan, and Soriano, *Closer to Liberation*; Diaz, *Postcolonial Configurations*; Velasco, *Queering the Global Filipina Body*.

33. Coll, *Remaking Citizenship*; Shah, "Understaffed and Overworked."

34. Cal/OSHA, "Voluntary Industry Guidelines to Protect the Health and Safety of Domestic Workers and Day Laborers."

WORKS CITED

Alba, Richard D. "Cohorts and the Dynamics of Ethnic Change." In *Social Structure and Human Lives*, edited by Matilda White Riley, 211–228. Beverly Hills, CA: Sage Publications, 1988.

Alvarez, Alvin N., and Linda P. Juang. "Filipino Americans and Racism: A Multiple Mediation Model of Coping." *Journal of Counseling Psychology* 57, no. 2 (2010): 167–178. https://doi.org/10.1037/a0019091.

Amorao, Amanda Solomon, Candice Custodio-Tan, and Jen Soriano, eds. *Closer to Liberation: Pin[a/x]y Activism in Theory and Practice*. Solana Beach, CA: Cognella Academic, 2023.

Armstrong, Pat, and Hugh Armstrong. *The Privatization of Care: The Case of Nursing Homes*. New York: Routledge, 2019.

Armstrong, Pat, Frode F. Jacobsen, Monique Lanoix, and Marta Szebehely. "The Crisis in the Nursing Home Labour Force: Where Is the Political Will?" In *Care Homes in a Turbulent Era: Do They Have a Future?*, edited by Pat Armstrong and Susan Braedley, 50–66. Northampton, MA: Edward Elgar Publishing, 2023.

Asis, Maruja M. B. "Repatriating Filipino Migrant Workers in the Time of the Pandemic." *Migration Research Series* 63 (2020).

Asis, Maruja Milagros B., Shirlena Huang, and Brenda S. A. Yeoh. "When the Light of the Home Is Abroad: Unskilled Female Migration and the Filipino Family." *Singapore Journal of Tropical Geography* 25, no. 2 (2004): 198–215. https://doi.org/10.1111/j.0129-7619.2004.00182.x.

Atienza, Paul Michael Leonardo. "The Promise of Intimacy: Gay Filipino Men on Mobile Digital Media in Manila and Los Angeles." PhD diss. University of Illinois at Urbana-Champaign, 2022.

Attal, Jordan Hannink, Ido Lurie, and Yehuda Neumark. "A Rapid Assessment of Migrant Careworkers' Psychosocial Status during Israel's COVID-19 Lockdown." *Israel*

Journal of Health Policy Research 9, no. 1 (2020): 1–11. https://doi.org/10.1186/s13584-020-00422-0.

Attias-Donfut, Claudine, and Joanne Cook. "Intergenerational Relationships in Migrant Families: Theoretical and Methodological Issues." In *Situating Children of Migrants across Borders and Origins*, edited by Laura Bernardi and Claudio Bolzman, 115–133. New York: Springer, 2017.

Ayalon, Liat. "Family and Family-Like Interactions in Households with Round-the-Clock Paid Foreign Carers in Israel." *Ageing & Society* 29, no. 5 (2009): 671–686. https://doi.org/10.1017/S0144686X09008393.

Baas, Michiel, and Brenda S. A. Yeoh. "Introduction: Migration Studies and Critical Temporalities." *Current Sociology* 67, no. 2 (2019): 161–168. https://doi.org/10.1177/0011392118792924.

Balce, Nerissa. *Body Parts of Empire: Visual Abjection, Filipino Images, and the American Archive*. Ann Arbor: University of Michigan Press, 2016.

Baldock, Cora Vellekoop. "Migrants and Their Parents: Caregiving from a Distance." *Journal of Family Issues* 21, no. 2 (2000): 205–224. https://journals.sagepub.com/doi/10.1177/019251300021002004.

Banta, Vanessa, and Geraldine Pratt. "Immobilised by the Pandemic: Filipino Domestic Workers and Seafarers in the Time of COVID-19." *Transactions of the Institute of British Geographers* 48, no. 3 (2023): 556–570. https://doi.org/10.1111/tran.12598.

Bautista, Mark, Antonio N. Martinez, and Dani O'Brien. "The Youth Will Speak: Youth Participatory Action Research as a Vehicle to Connect an Ethnic Studies Pedagogy to Communities." In *"White" Washing American Education: The New Culture Wars in Ethnic Studies*, edited by Denise M. Sandoval, Anthony J. Ratcliff, Tracy Lachica Buenavista, and James R. Marín, 97–115. New York: Praeger, 2016.

Beneria, Lourdes. "The Enduring Debate over Unpaid Labour." *International Labour Review* 138, no. 3 (1999): 287–309. https://doi.org/10.1111/j.1564-913X.1999.tb00389.x.

Bezanson, Kate, and Meg Luxton. *Social Reproduction: Feminist Political Economy Challenges Neo-Liberalism*. Montreal: McGill-Queen's University Press, 2006.

Bhattacharya, Tithi, ed. *Social Reproduction Theory: Remapping Class, Recentering Oppression*. London: Pluto Press, 2017.

Billies, Michelle, Valerie Francisco, Patricia Krueger, and Darla Linville. "Participatory Action Research: Our Methodological Roots." *International Review of Qualitative Research* 3, no. 3 (2010): 277–286. https://doi.org/10.1525/irqr.2010.3.3.277.

Bismark, Marie, Karen Willis, Sophie Lewis, and Natasha Smallwood. *Experiences of Health Workers in the COVID-19 Pandemic: In Their Own Words*. New York: Routledge, 2022.

Bonus, Rick. *Locating Filipino Americans: Ethnicity and the Cultural Politics of Space*. Philadelphia: Temple University Press, 2000.

Bonus, Rick, and Antonio Tiongson Jr. *Filipinx American Studies: Reckoning, Reclamation, Transformation.* New York: Fordham University Press, 2022.

Boris, Eileen, and Jennifer Klein. *Caring for America: Home Health Workers in the Shadow of the Welfare State.* New York: Oxford University Press, 2015.

Boris, Eileen, and Jennifer Klein. "Frontline Caregivers: Still Struggling." *Dissent* 59, no. 1 (2012): 46–50. https://doi.org/10.1353/dss.2012.0020.

Brabeck, Kalina, M. Lykes, and Rachel Hershberg. "Framing Immigration to and Deportation from the United States: Guatemalan and Salvadoran Families Make Meaning of Their Experiences." *Faculty Publications*, 2011, March. http://digitalcommons.ric.edu/facultypublications/263.

Braedley, Susan, Prince Owusu, Anna Przednowek, and Pat Armstrong. "We're Told, 'Suck It Up': Long-Term Care Workers' Psychological Health and Safety." *Ageing International* 43, no. 1 (2018): 91–109. https://doi.org/10.1007/s12126-017-9288-4.

Brennan, Deborah, Bettina Cass, Susan Himmelweit, and Marta Szebehely. "The Marketisation of Care: Rationales and Consequences in Nordic and Liberal Care Regimes." *Journal of European Social Policy* 22, no. 4 (2012): 377–391. https://doi.org/10.1177/0958928712449772.

Browne, Colette V., Kathryn L. Braun, and Pam Arnsberger. "Filipinas as Residential Long-Term Care Providers: Influence of Cultural Values, Structural Inequity, and Immigrant Status on Choosing This Work." *Journal of Gerontological Social Work* 48, nos. 3–4 (2006): 439–455. https://doi.org/10.1300/j083v48n03_10.

Bryceson, Deborah, and Ulla Vuorela, eds. *The Transnational Family: New European Frontiers and Global Networks.* New York: Routledge, 2020.

Buenavista, Tracy Lachica, Uma M. Jayakumar, and Kimberly Misa. "Contextualizing Asian American Education through Critical Race Theory: An Example of U.S. Pilipino College Student Experiences." *New Directions for Institutional Research* 2009, no. 142: 69–81. http://doi.org/10.1002/ir.297.

Burns, Lucy Mae San Pablo. "Masagana 99: Beyond Seeds, Grains, and Stalks." *Alon: Journal for Filipinx American and Diasporic Studies* 1, no. 3 (2021). https://doi.org/10.5070/LN41355442.

Caballero, Jennifer, Nancy Dayne, Wendy Reiboldt, and Lana Tran. "'It's the Filipino Way': Remittance Practices of Filipino American Families." *Journal of Family & Consumer Sciences* 113, no. 1 (2021). http://doi.org/10.14307/JFCS113.1.40.

Cabalquinto, Earvin Charles. "Ambivalent Intimacies: Entangled Pains and Gains through Facebook Use in Transnational Family Life." In *Digital Intimate Publics and Social Media*, edited by Amy Shields Dobson, Brady Robards, and Nicholas Carah, 247–263. New York: Palgrave Macmillan, 2018.

Cabalquinto, Earvin Charles B. *(Im)mobile Homes: Family Life at a Distance in the Age of Mobile Media.* New York: Oxford University Press, 2022.

Cabalquinto, Earvin Charles B. "'We're Not Only Here but We're There in Spirit': Asymmetrical Mobile Intimacy and the Transnational Filipino Family." *Mobile Media & Communication* 6, no. 1 (2018): 37–52. https://doi.org/10.1177/2050157917722055.

Cahill, Caitlin. "'Why Do They Hate Us?' Reframing Immigration through Participatory Action Research." *Area* 42, no. 2 (2010): 152–161.

Cal/OSHA. "Voluntary Industry Guidelines to Protect the Health and Safety of Domestic Workers and Day Laborers." 2022. https://www.dir.ca.gov/dosh/documents/Voluntary-Industry-Guidelines-SB-321.pdf.

Cammarota, Julio, and Michelle Fine. *Revolutionizing Education: Youth Participatory Action Research in Motion*. New York: Routledge, 2008.

Castaneda, Michael Schulze-Oechtering, and Wayne Jopanda. "Transpacific Freedom Dreams: The Radical Legacy of Silme Domingo and Gene Viernes." In *Filipino American Transnational Activism*, edited by Robyn M. Rodriguez, 227–247. Leiden, The Netherlands: Brill, 2019.

Chang, Grace. *Disposable Domestics: Immigrant Women Workers in the Global Economy*. Boston: South End Press, 2000.

Chin, Gabriel J., and Rose Cuison Villazor. *The Immigration and Nationality Act of 1965: Legislating a New America*. New York: Cambridge University Press, 2015.

Choudhry, U. K., Surinder Jandu, J. Mahal, R. Singh, H. Sohi-Pabla, and B. Mutta. "Health Promotion and Participatory Action Research with South Asian Women." *Journal of Nursing Scholarship: An Official Publication of Sigma Theta Tau International Honor Society of Nursing / Sigma Theta Tau* 34, no. 1 (2002): 75–81. https://doi.org/10.1111/j.1547-5069.2002.00075.x.

Chowdhury, Reshmi, and Gloria Gutman. "Migrant Live-In Caregivers Providing Care to Canadian Older Adults: An Exploratory Study of Workers' Life and Job Satisfaction." *Journal of Population Ageing* 5, no. 4 (2012): 215–240. https://doi.org/10.1007/s12062-012-9073-9.

Choy, Catherine Ceniza. *Empire of Care: Nursing and Migration in Filipino American History*. Durham: Duke University Press, 2003.

Clergé, Orly. *The New Noir: Race, Identity, and Diaspora in Black Suburbia*. Berkeley: University of California Press, 2019.

Colen, Shellee. "Stratified Reproduction and West Indian Childcare Workers and Employers in New York." In *Feminist Anthropology: A Reader*, edited by Ellen Lewin, 380–396. Malden, MA: Blackwell, 2009.

Coll, Kathleen. *Remaking Citizenship: Latina Immigrants and the New American Politics*. Stanford: Stanford University Press, 2010.

Coll, Kathleen Marie, Juana Flores, María Jiménez, Nathalie López, Andrea Lauren Lee, Maria Carrillo, Laura Camberos, et al. "It's a Matter of Trust: How Thirty

Years of History Prepared a Community-Based Organization to Respond to the COVID-19 Pandemic." *Social Sciences* 12, no. 8 (2023): 423.

Collie, Philippa, James Liu, Astrid Podsiadlowski, and Sara Kindon. "You Can't Clap with One Hand: Learnings to Promote Culturally Grounded Participatory Action Research with Migrant and Former Refugee Communities." *International Journal of Intercultural Relations* 34, no. 2 (2010): 141–149. https://doi.org/10.1016/j.ijintrel.2009.11.008.

Colting-Stol, Jacqueline. "How Mutual Aid and Community Care Ignite Further Grassroots Organizing Possibilities for Long-Term Change: Reflections from the Case of Kapit-Bisig Laban COVID Montreal (Linked Arms in the Struggle against Covid)." *Alon: Journal for Filipinx American and Diasporic Studies* 2, no. 2 (2022). https://doi.org/10.5070/LN42258019.

Cranford, Cynthia J. *Home Care Fault Lines: Understanding Tensions and Creating Alliances*. Ithaca: Cornell University Press, 2020.

Cranford, Cynthia J., and Jennifer Jihye Chun. "Multi-level Analyses of Homecare Labor." In *Research Handbook on Intersectionality*, edited by Mary Romero, 385–403. Northampton, MA: Edgar Elver Publishing, 2023.

Cristancho, Sergio, D. Marcela Garces, Karen E. Peters, and Benjamin C. Mueller. "Listening to Rural Hispanic Immigrants in the Midwest: A Community-Based Participatory Assessment of Major Barriers to Health Care Access and Use." *Qualitative Health Research* 18, no. 5 (2008): 633–646. https://doi.org/10.1177/1049732308316669.

Critical Filipino Studies Collective. "Anti–Martial Law Syllabus." *Alon: Journal for Filipinx American and Diasporic Studies* 2, no. 2 (2022). https://doi.org/10.5070/LN42258009.

Curammeng, Edward R., and Allyson Tintiangco-Cubales. "Growing Our Own Hope: The Development of a Pin@ y Teacher Pipeline." In *Confronting Racism in Teacher Education*, edited by Bree Picower and Rita Kohli, 157–163. New York: Routledge, 2017.

Dalla Costa, Mariarosa. "Capitalism and Reproduction." *Open Marxism* 3 (1995): 7–16.

Datu, Jesus Alfonso D., and Frank D. Fincham. "The Relational and Mental Health Payoffs of Staying Gritty during the COVID-19 Pandemic: A Cross-Cultural Study in the Philippines and the United States." *Journal of Social and Personal Relationships* 39, no. 3 (2022): 459–480. https://doi.org/10.1177/02654075211029380.

Daus-Magbual, Arlene, Roderick Daus-Magbual, and Allyson Tintiangco-Cubales. "Pin@ y Educational PARtnerships: Ethnic Studies Students, Teachers and Leaders as Scholar Activists." *AAPI Nexus: Policy, Practice, and Community* 16, nos. 1–2 (2019). https://doi.org/10.36650/nexus16.1-2_220-244_Daus-Magbual2Tintiango-Cubales.

David, Eric John Ramos. *Brown Skin, White Minds: Filipino- / American Postcolonial Psychology*. Charlotte, NC: Information Age Publishing, 2013.

David, E. J. R., Dinghy Kristine B. Sharma, and Jessica Petalio. "Losing Kapwa: Colonial Legacies and the Filipino American Family." *Asian American Journal of Psychology, Moving beyond the Model Minority* 8, no. 1 (2017): 43–55. https://doi.org/10.1037/aap0000068.

Davis, Angela Y. *Women, Race & Class.* New York: Vintage, 1983.

Day, Iyko. *Alien Capital: Asian Racialization and the Logic of Settler Colonial Capitalism.* Durham: Duke University Press, 2016.

de Borja, Jean Aaron. "Overseas Filipino Workers and the COVID-19 Pandemic: Exploring the Emotional Labor of Persistence." *Emotion, Space and Society* 41 (2021): 100838. https://doi.org/10.1016/j.emospa.2021.100838.

De Castro, A. B., Gilbert C. Gee, and David T. Takeuchi. "Job-Related Stress and Chronic Health Conditions among Filipino Immigrants." *Journal of Immigrant and Minority Health* 10 (2008): 551–558. https://doi.org/10.1007/s10903-008-9138-2.

De Castro, Arnold B., Gilbert C. Gee, and David T. Takeuchi. "Workplace Discrimination and Health among Filipinos in the United States." *American Journal of Public Health* 98, no. 3 (2008): 520–526. https://doi.org/10.2105/AJPH.2007.110163.

de Leon, Conely. "'Pagod, Dugot, Pawis (Exhaustion, Blood, and Sweat)': Transnational Practices of Care and Emotional Labour among Filipino Kin Networks." PhD diss. York University, Toronto, Ontario, 2018.

de Leon, Conely, and Pahinga Collective. "A Call to Rest: Pahinga as Resistance and Refusal." *Alon: Journal for Filipinx American and Diasporic Studies* 2, no. 2 (2022). https://doi.org/10.5070/LN42258015.

De Tona, Carla, Annalisa Frisina, and Deianira Ganga. "Editorial: Research Methods in Ethnic and Migration Studies." *Migration Letters* 7, no. 1 (2010): 1–6.

Del Vecchio, Deanna, Nisha Toomey, and Eve Tuck. "Placing Photovoice: Participatory Action Research with Undocumented Migrant Youth in the Hudson Valley." *Critical Questions in Education* 8, no. 4 (2017): 358–376. https://doi.org/10.1177%2F14733250211039510.

Delgado, Daniela. 2017. "The Health Impacts of Domestic Labor on Women Workers in Massachusetts." PhD diss. Harvard University.

Diaz, Josen Masangkay. *Postcolonial Configurations: Dictatorship, the Racial Cold War, and Filipino America.* Durham: Duke University Press, 2022.

Dill, LeConté J., Shavaun S. Sutton, Emily S. Cowan, and Arielsela Holdbrook-Smith. "Oh, We Got Beef?! Ruptures, Refusals, Rifts, and Re-Commitments in Academic–Community Partnerships." *Departures in Critical Qualitative Research* 11, no. 3 (2022): 40–56. https://doi.org/10.1525/dcqr.2022.11.3.40.

Dilworth-Anderson, Peggye, Sharon W. Williams, and Theresa Cooper. "The Contexts of Experiencing Emotional Distress among Family Caregivers to Elderly African Americans." *Family Relations* 48, no. 4 (1999): 391–396. https://doi.org/10.2307/585246.

Duffy, Mignon. "Doing the Dirty Work: Gender, Race, and Reproductive Labor in Historical Perspective." *Gender & Society* 21, no. 3 (2007): 313–336. https://doi.org/10.1177/0891243207300764.

Dutta, Mohan J., Sarah Comer, Daniel Teo, Pauline Luk, Mary Lee, Dazzelyn Zapata, Arudhra Krishnaswamy, and Satveer Kaur. "Health Meanings among Foreign Domestic Workers in Singapore: A Culture-Centered Approach." *Health Communication* 33, no. 5 (2018): 643–652. https://doi.org/10.1080/10410236.2017.1292576.

Eidelson, Josh. "Nurses Who Faced Lawsuits for Quitting Are Fighting Back." Bloomberg.com, February 22, 2022. https://www.bloomberg.com/news/features/2022-02-02/underpaid-contract-nurses-who-faced-fines-lawsuits-for-quitting-fight-back.

England, Paula. "Emerging Theories of Care Work." *Annual Review of Sociology* 31 (2005): 381–399. https://doi.org/10.1146/annurev.soc.31.041304.122317.

Enriquez, Virgilio. *From Colonial to Liberation Psychology: The Philippine Experience*. Quezon City: University of the Philippines Press, 2013.

Escobedo, Loraine A., Brittany N. Morey, and Ninez A. Ponce. "Lost on the Frontline, and Lost in the Data: COVID-19 Deaths among Filipinx Healthcare Workers in the United States." SSRN Scholarly Paper. 2021. https://doi.org/10.2139/ssrn.3792198.

Espia, Juhn Chris P., Alice Prieto-Carolino, Liberty N. Espectato, and Ruby Napata. "Into the Unknown: Migration and the Politics of Identity in Four Coastal Municipalities in Southwest Panay, Philippines." *Ocean & Coastal Management* 211 (2021): 105801. https://doi.org/10.1016/j.ocecoaman.2021.105801.

Espiritu, Augusto. "Transnationalism and Filipino American Historiography." *Journal of Asian American Studies* 11, no. 2 (2008): 171–184. https://doi.org/10.1353/jaas.0.0005.

Espiritu, Yen Le. *Home Bound: Filipino American Lives across Cultures, Communities, and Countries*. Berkeley: University of California Press, 2003.

Faul, Anna C., Tara J. Schapmire, Joseph D'Ambrosio, Dennis Feaster, C. Shawn Oak, and Amanda Farley. "Promoting Sustainability in Frontline Home Care Aides: Understanding Factors Affecting Job Retention in the Home Care Workforce." *Home Health Care Management & Practice* 22, no. 6 (2010): 408–416. https://doi.org/10.1177/1084822309348896.

Federici, Silvia. "Social Reproduction Theory: History, Issues, and Present Challenges." *Radical Philosophy* 204 (2019): 55–57.

Federici, Silvia. *Wages against Housework*. Bristol, UK: Falling Wall Press, 1975.

Fernandez, Ica, Justin Muyot, Abbey Pangilinan, and Nastassja Quijano. "A Hero's Welcome? Repatriated Overseas Filipino Workers and COVID-19." *LSE Southeast Asia* (blog) (2020). https://blogs.lse.ac.uk/seac/2020/10/08/a-heros-welcome-repatriated-overseas-filipino-workers-and-covid-19.

Ferrera, Maria J. "The Transformative Impact of Cultural Portals on the Ethnic Identity

Development of Second-Generation Filipino-American Emerging Adults." *Journal of Ethnic & Cultural Diversity in Social Work* 26, no. 3 (2017): 236–253. https://doi.org/10.1080/15313204.2016.1141739.

Fields, Jessica. *Risky Lessons: Sex Education and Social Inequality*. New Brunswick: Rutgers University Press, 2008.

Fine, Michelle, and María Elena Torre. "Intimate Details." *Action Research* 4, no. 3 (2006): 253–269. https://doi.org/10.1177/1476750306066801.

Folbre, Nancy. *The Invisible Heart: Economics and Family Values*. New York: New Press, 2002.

Francisco, Valerie. "Accumulating Delay: Filipino Time, COVID-19 and Experiences of Male Returnees in Cebu." *Asia Pacific Migration Journal*. Forthcoming.

———. "'Ang Ating Iisang Kuwento': Our Collective Story: Migrant Filipino Workers and Participatory Action Research." *Action Research* 12, no. 1 (2014): 78–93. https://psycnet.apa.org/doi/10.1177/1476750313515283.

———. "From Where I Sit." *International Review of Qualitative Research* 3, no. 3 (2010): 287–310.

———. "'The Internet Is Magic': Technology, Intimacy, and Transnational Families." *Critical Sociology* 41, no. 1 (2013): 173–190. https://doi.org/10.1177/0896920513484602.

———. "Kuwentuhan as a Method." In *Handbook of Social Inclusion: Research and Practices in Health and Social Sciences*, edited by Pranee Liamputtong, 1–23. Cham, Switzerland: Springer International Publishing, 2020. https://doi.org/10.1007/978-3-030-48277-0_83-1.

———. *The Labor of Care: Filipina Migrants and Transnational Families in the Digital Age*. Urbana: University of Illinois Press, 2018.

———. "Migrante, Abante: Building Filipino Migrant Worker Leadership through Participatory Action Research." In *Just Work? Migrant Workers' Struggles Today*, edited by Aziz Choudry and Mondli Hlatshwayo, 211–229. London: Pluto Press, 2016.

Francisco-Menchavez, Valerie, and Edwin Carlos. "Kuwentuhan across Generations: Intergenerational Participatory Methods in Exploring Filipino Immigrant and Filipino American Transnational Experiences." In *The Routledge International Handbook of Critical Participatory Inquiry in Transnational Research Contexts*, edited by Giovanni Dazzo, Meagan Call-Cummings, and Melissa Hauber-Özer, 238-249. New York: Routledge, 2023.

Francisco-Menchavez, Valerie, Elaika Celemen, and Kristal Osorio. "Filipino Formal Caregivers to the Elderly and Normalized Exploitation in the Workplace." *Alon: Journal for Filipinx American and Diasporic Studies* 1, no. 1 (2021): 51–67. https://doi.org/10.5070/LN41149607.

Francisco-Menchavez, Valerie, Jessa Delos Reyes, Tiffany Mendoza, Stephanie

Ancheta, and Katrina Liwanag. "Claiming Kapwa: Filipino Immigrants, Community-Based Organizations, and Community Citizenship in San Francisco." *New Political Science* 40, no. 2 (2018): 404–417.

Francisco, Valerie, and Robyn Rodriguez. "Coming to America: The Business of Trafficked Workers." In *The Immigration and Nationality Act of 1965: Legislating a New America*, edited by Gabriel J. Chin and Rose Cuison Villazor, 273–291. New York: Cambridge University Press, 2015.

Francisco-Menchavez, Valerie, and Ethel Tungohan. "Mula sa masa, tungo sa masa, From the People, to the People: Building Migrant Worker Power through Participatory Action Research." *Migration Letters* 17, no. 2 (2020): 257–264. https://doi.org/10.33182/ml.v17i2.768.

Fraser, Nancy. "Capitalism's Crisis of Care." *Dissent* 63, no. 4 (2016): 30–37. https://doi.org/10.1353/dss.2016.0071.

Fukushima, Annie Isabel. "An American Haunting: Unsettling Witnessing in Transnational Migration, the Ghost Case, and Human Trafficking." *Feminist Formations* 28, no. 1 (2016): 146–165. https://www.jstor.org/stable/44508117.

Fukushima, Annie Isabel. *Migrant Crossings: Witnessing Human Trafficking in the US*. Stanford: Stanford University Press, 2019.

Galam, Roderick. "Futures on Hold: The Covid-19 Pandemic, International Seafaring, and the Immobility of Aspiring Filipino Seafarers." *LSE Southeast Asia* (blog), September 22, 2020. https://blogs.lse.ac.uk/seac/2020/09/22/futures-on-hold.

Geraci, Angela Ann, Barbara Hutchison, and Ardith R. Brunt. "California's Newly Reformed Residential Care Facilities for the Elderly." *California Journal of Politics and Policy* 7, no. 2 (2015): 1–14.

Gilmore, Ruth Wilson. *Abolition Geography: Essays towards Liberation*. New York: Verso Books, 2022.

———. "Fatal Couplings of Power and Difference: Notes on Racism and Geography." *Professional Geographer* 54, no. 1 (2002): 15–24. https://doi.org/10.1111/0033-0124.00310.

Giordano, Chiara. "Freedom or Money? The Dilemma of Migrant Live-In Elderly Carers in Times of COVID-19." *Gender, Work & Organization* 28, no. S1 (2021): 137–150. https://doi.org/10.1111/gwao.12509.

Glenn, Evelyn Nakano. "From Servitude to Service Work: Historical Continuities in the Racial Division of Paid Reproductive Labor." *Signs* 18, no. 1 (1992): 1–43.

Glenn, Evelyn Nakano. "Racial Ethnic Women's Labor: The Intersection of Race, Gender, and Class Oppression." *Review of Radical Political Economics* 17, no. 3 (1985): 86–108. https://doi.org/10.1177/048661348501700306.

Gonzalves, Theodore S., and Roderick N. Labrador. *Filipinos in Hawai'i*. Mount Pleasant, SC: Arcadia Publishing, 2011.

Gordon, Judith R., Rachel A. Pruchno, Maureen Wilson-Genderson, Wendy Marcinkus Murphy, and Miriam Rose. "Balancing Caregiving and Work: Role Conflict and Role Strain Dynamics." *Journal of Family Issues* 33, no. 5 (2012): 662–689. https://doi.org/10.1177/0192513X11425322.

Guevarra, Anna Romina. "The Balikbayan Researcher: Negotiating Vulnerability in Fieldwork with Filipino Labor Brokers." *Journal of Contemporary Ethnography* 35, no. 5 (2006): 526–551. https://doi.org/10.1177/0891241605285116.

Guevarra, Anna Romina. *Marketing Dreams, Manufacturing Heroes: The Transnational Labor.* New Brunswick: Rutgers University Press, 2009.

Guglielmo, Jennifer, and Michelle Joffroy. "A History of Domestic Work and Worker Organizing." 2020. https://www.dwherstories.com.

Guishard, Monique. "The False Paths, the Endless Labors, the Turns Now This Way and Now That: Participatory Action Research, Mutual Vulnerability, and the Politics of Inquiry." *Urban Review* 41, no. 1 (2009): 85–105. https://doi.org/10.1007/s11256-008-0096-8.

Guishard, Monique Antoinette, Alexis Halkovic, Anne Galletta, and Peiwei Li. "Toward Epistemological Ethics: Centering Communities and Social Justice in Qualitative Research." *Forum Qualitative Sozialforschung/Forum: Qualitative Social Research* 19, no. 3 (2018). https://doi.org/10.17169/fqs-19.3.3145.

Guishard, Monique A., Devin A. Heyward, Justin T. Brown, and Marcia Stoddard-Pennant. "What We Not Finna Do: Respectfully Collaborating with Skinfolk and Kinfolk in Black Feminist Participatory Action Research." *Global Journal of Community Psychology Practice* 12, no. 2 (2021): 1–36.

Gutierrez, Armand. "Being Filipino without the Philippines: Second-Generation Filipino American Ethnic Identification." In *Filipino American Transnational Activism*, edited by Robyn M. Rodriguez, 26–53. New York: Brill, 2019.

———. "A Family Affair: How and Why Second-Generation Filipino-Americans Engage in Transnational Social and Economic Connections." *Ethnic and Racial Studies* 41, no. 2 (2018): 229–247. https://doi.org/10.1080/01419870.2017.1287418.

———. "Mediated Remittances: Transnational Economic Contributions from Second-Generation Filipino Americans." *Global Networks* 18, no. 3 (2018): 523–540. https://doi.org/10.1111/glob.12198.

Gutierrez, Rose Ann, H. Piñon, and M. T. Valmocena. "Co-Creating Knowledge with Undocumented Filipino Students: Kuwentuhan as Research Method." *New Directions for Higher Education.* December 8, 2023 (203): 77–92. http://doi.org/10.1002/he.20478.

Harrington, Charlene, and Frode F. Jacobsen. "Nurse Staffing in Nursing Homes in Industrialized Countries." In *The Privatization of Care: The Case of Nursing Homes*, edited by Pat Armstrong and Hugh Armstrong, 177–195. New York: Routledge, 2019.

Harrington, Charlene, Allyson M. Pollock, Shailen Sutaria. "Privatization of Nursing Homes in the United Kingdom and the United States." In *The Privatization of Care: The Case of Nursing Homes*, edited by Pat Armstrong and Hugh Armstrong, 51–67. New York: Routledge, 2019.

Hobart, Hi'ilei Julia Kawehipuaakahaopulani, and Tamara Kneese. "Radical Care: Survival Strategies for Uncertain Times." *Social Text* 38, no. 1 (2020): 1–16. https://doi.org/10.1215/01642472-7971067.

Hochschild, Arlie Russell. *The Managed Heart: Commercialization of Human Feeling*. Berkeley: University of California Press, 2003.

Hossfeld, Karen J. "Hiring Immigrant Women: Silicon Valley's 'Simple Formula.'" In *Race and Ethnic Conflict: Contending Views on Prejudice, Discrimination, and Ethnoviolence*, edited by Fred L. Pincus and Howard J. Ehrlich, 162–179. New York: Routledge, 2019.

Huang, Shirlena, Brenda S. A. Yeoh, and Mitoka Toyota. "Caring for the Elderly: The Embodied Labour of Migrant Care Workers in Singapore." *Global Networks* 12, no. 2 (2012): 195–215. https://doi.org/10.1111/j.1471-0374.2012.00347.x.

IBON Foundation. *IBON Manual on Facilitating Participatory Research*. Quezon City, Philippines: IBON Foundation, 2004.

Iecovich, Esther. "What Makes Migrant Live-In Home Care Workers in Elder Care Be Satisfied with Their Job?" *The Gerontologist* 51, no. 5 (2011): 617–629. https://doi.org/10.1093/geront/gnr048.

International Organization for Migration. "COVID-19 Impact Assessment on Returned Overseas Filipino Workers." 2021. https://dtm.iom.int/reports/philippines-%E2%80%93-covid-19-impact-assessment-returned-overseas-filipino-workers-may-2021.

Isaac, Allan Punzalan. *Filipino Time: Affective Worlds and Contracted Labor*. New York: Fordham University Press, 2021.

Jeung, R., and K. Nham. "Incidents of Coronavirus-Related Discrimination." 2020. http://www.asianpacificpolicyandplanningcouncil.org/wpcontent/uploads/STOP_AAP_HATE_MONTHLY_REPORT_4_23_20.pdf.

Jocson, Korina M. "Whose Story Is It Anyway? Teaching Social Studies and Making Use of Kuwento." *Multicultural Perspectives* 11, no. 1 (2009): 31–36. https://doi.org/10.1080/15210960902717445.

Jopanda, Wayne. "Talk Story Methodologies (Kuwentuhan) Kuwentuhan." In *Bloomsbury Encyclopedia of Social Justice in Education*, Vol. 6: *Language, Literacy, Youth and Culture*, edited by Arturo Cortez and José Lizarraga. Bloomsbury Publishing (2025).

Kahakalau, Kū. "Indigenous Heuristic Action Research: Bridging Western and Indigenous Research Methodologies." *Hulili: Multidisciplinary Research on Hawaiian Well-Being* 1, no. 1 (2004): 19–33.

Kang, Jong Woo, and Ma Concepcion Latoja. "COVID-19 and Overseas Filipino Workers: Return Migration and Reintegration into the Home Country—the Philippine Case." *Asian Development Bank*, 2022.

Kang, Miliann. *The Managed Hand: Race, Gender, and the Body in Beauty Service Work.* Berkeley: University of California Press, 2010.

Kares, Faith R. "Practicing 'Enlightened Capitalism': 'Fil-Am' Heroes, NGO Activism, and the Reconstitution of Class Difference in the Philippines." *Philippine Studies: Historical and Ethnographic Viewpoints* 62, no. 2 (2014): 175–204. http://dx.doi.org/10.1353/phs.2014.0011.

Kodama, Corinne M., and Rhonda Laylo. "The Unique Context of Identity-Based Student Organizations in Developing Leadership." *New Directions for Student Leadership* 2017, no. 155 (2017): 71–81. https://doi.org/10.1002/yd.20251.

Kofman, Eleonore. 2012. "Rethinking Care through Social Reproduction: Articulating Circuits of Migration." *Social Politics: International Studies in Gender, State & Society* 19, no. 1: 142–162. https://doi.org/10.1093/sp/jxr030.

Krueger-Henney, Patricia. "Through Space into the Flesh: Mapping Inscriptions of Anti-Black Racist and Ableist Schooling on Young People's Bodies." In *Disability as Meta Curriculum*, edited by Gillian Parekh, Elizabeth J. Grace, and Nirmala Erevelles, 70–85. New York: Routledge, 2023.

———. "What Are We Listening For? (Participatory Action) Research and Embodied Social Listening to the Permanence of Anti-Black Racism in Education." *International Journal of Critical Pedagogy* 7, no. 3 (2016).

Krueger-Henney, Patricia, and Jessica Ruglis. "PAR Is a Way of Life: Participatory Action Research as Core Re-Training for Fugitive Research Praxis." *Educational Philosophy and Theory* 52, no. 9 (2020): 961–972. https://doi.org/10.1080/00131857.2020.1762569.

Lan, Pei-Chia. "Shifting Borders and Migrant Workers' Im/Mobility: The Case of Taiwan during the COVID-19 Pandemic." *Asian and Pacific Migration Journal* 31, no. 3 (2022): 225–246. https://doi.org/10.1177/01171968221127495.

Laslett, Barbara, and Johanna Brenner. "Gender and Social Reproduction: Historical Perspectives." *Annual Review of Sociology* 15, no. 1 (1989): 381–404. https://www.jstor.org/stable/2083231.

Levitt, Peggy, and Mary C. Waters. *The Changing Face of Home: The Transnational Lives of the Second Generation.* New York: Russell Sage Foundation, 2002.

Li, Yan, and Sandro Galea. "Racism and the COVID-19 Epidemic: Recommendations for Health Care Workers." *American Journal of Public Health* 110, no. 7 (2020): 956–957. https://doi.org/10.2105/AJPH.2020.305698.

Lindio-McGovern, Ligaya, and Isidor Wallimann. *Globalization and Third World Women: Exploitation, Coping, and Resistance.* New York: Routledge, 2016.

Litam, Stacey Diane Aranez, and Seungbin Oh. "Coping Strategies as Moderators of COVID-19 Racial Discrimination in Filipino Americans." *Asian American Journal of Psychology* 13, no. 1 (2022): 18–29. https://doi.org/10.1037/aap0000253.

Lowe, Lisa. *Immigrant Acts: On Asian American Cultural Politics*. Durham: Duke University Press, 1996.

Mabalon, Dawn Bohulano. *Little Manila Is in the Heart: The Making of the Filipina/o American Community in Stockton, California*. Durham: Duke University Press, 2013.

Macdonald, Fiona, and Sara Charlesworth. "Cash for Care under the NDIS: Shaping Care Workers' Working Conditions?" *Journal of Industrial Relations* 58, no. 5 (2016): 627–646. https://doi.org/10.1177/0022185615623083.

Madriz, Esther I. "Using Focus Groups with Lower Socioeconomic Status Latina Women." *Qualitative Inquiry* 4, no. 1 (1998): 114–128. https://doi.org/10.1177/107780049800400107.

Maramba, Dina C., and Samuel D. Museus. "The Utility of Using Mixed-Methods and Intersectionality Approaches in Conducting Research on Filipino American Students' Experiences with the Campus Climate and on Sense of Belonging." *New Directions for Institutional Research* 2011, no. 151 (2011): 93–101. https://doi.org/10.1002/ir.401.

Mata-Codesal, Diana, Laure Kloetzer, and Concepción Maiztegui-Oñate. "Strengths, Risks, and Limits of Doing Participatory Research in Migration Studies." *Migration Letters* 17, no. 2 (2020): 201–210. https://doi.org/10.33182/ml.v17i2.934.

McCarthy, Brendan. 2013. "In Depth: Pipeline of Alleged Human Trafficking from Philippines to the Gulf." https://www.wwltv.com/article/news/in-depth-pipeline-of-alleged-human-trafficking-from-philippines-to-the-gulf/289-320078017.

Meyer, Mechthild C., Sara Torres, Nubia Cermeño, Lynne MacLean, and Rosa Monzón. "Immigrant Women Implementing Participatory Research in Health Promotion." *Western Journal of Nursing Research* 25, no. 7 (2003): 815–834. https://doi.org/10.1177/0193945903256707.

Minkler, Meredith, Pam Tau Lee, Alex Tom, Charlotte Chang, Alvaro Morales, Shaw San Liu, Alicia Salvatore, et al. "Using Community-Based Participatory Research to Design and Initiate a Study on Immigrant Worker Health and Safety in San Francisco's Chinatown Restaurants." *American Journal of Industrial Medicine* 53, no. 4 (2010): 361–371. https://doi.org/10.1002/ajim.20791.

Mitchell, Tania D., and Kathleen M. Coll. "Ethnic Studies as a Site for Political Education: Critical Service Learning and the California Domestic Worker Bill of Rights." *PS: Political Science & Politics* 50, no. 1 (2017): 187–192. https://doi.org/10.1017/S1049096516002419.

Montero-Sieburth, Martha Adelia. "Who Gives 'Voice' or 'Empowers Migrants' in Participatory Action Research? Challenges and Solutions." *Migration Letters* 17, no. 2 (2020): 1–8. https://doi.org/10.33182/ml.v17i2.806.

Nadasen, Premilla. *Care: The Highest Stage of Capitalism*. Chicago: Haymarket Books, 2023.

———. "Citizenship Rights, Domestic Work, and the Fair Labor Standards Act." *Journal of Policy History* 24, no. 1 (2012): 74–94. https://doi.org/10.1017/S0898030611000388.

———. *Household Workers Unite: The Untold Story of African American Women Who Built a Movement*. Boston: Beacon Press, 2015.

Nasol, Katherine. "The Governance of Care." PhD diss. University of California, Davis, 2023.

Nasol, Katherine, and Valerie Francisco-Menchavez. "Filipino Home Care Workers: Invisible Frontline Workers in the COVID-19 Crisis in the United States." *American Behavioral Scientist* 65, no. 10 (2021): 1365–1383. https://doi.org/10.1177/00027642211000410.

Navarro, Vicente. "The Labor Process and Health: A Historical Materialist Interpretation." *International Journal of Health Services* 12, no. 1 (1982): 5–29. https://www.jstor.org/stable/45130032.

Nazareno, Jennifer. "Welfare State Replacements: Deinstitutionalization, Privatization, and the Outsourcing to Immigrant Women Enterprise." *International Journal of Health Services* 48, no. 2 (2018): 247–266. https://doi.org/10.1177/0020731418759876.

Nazareno, Jennifer Pabelonia, Rhacel Salazar Parreñas, and Yu-Kang Fan. "Can I Ever Retire? The Plight of Migrant Filipino Elderly Caregivers in Los Angeles." *UCLA: Institute for Research on Labor and Employment*, 2014.

Nishida, Akemi. *Just Care: Messy Entanglements of Disability, Dependency, and Desire*. Philadelphia: Temple University Press, 2022.

Occupational Safety and Health Administration (OSHA). "Guidelines for Nursing Homes." 2009. https://www.osha.gov/sites/default/files/publications/final_nh_guidelines.pdf.

Oliva-Arocas, Adriana, Pierina Benavente, Elena Ronda, and Esperanza Diaz. "Health of International Migrant Workers during the COVID-19 Pandemic: A Scoping Review." *Frontiers in Public Health* 10 (2022). https://www.frontiersin.org/articles/10.3389/fpubh.2022.816597.

Ong, Josephine. "Care as Collective Revolution: Filipino Women's Activist Histories and Contemporary Solidarities in Guåhan." *Alon: Journal for Filipinx American and Diasporic Studies* 2, no. 2 (2022). https://doi.org/10.5070/LN42258018.

Orteza, Grace O. *Pakikipagkuwentuhan: Isang Pamamaraan Ng Sama-Samang Pananalik- Sik, Pagpapatotoo, at Pagtulong Sa Sikolohiyang Pilipino [Pakikipagkuwentuhan: A Method of Collective Research, Establishing Validity, and Contributing to Filipino Psychology]*. PPRTH Occasional Papers Series, Philippine Psychology Research and Training House, 1997.

Ortiga, Yasmin Y., and Karen Anne S. Liao. "When a Pandemic Disrupts the Export of People." *Research Collection School of Social Sciences*, Paper 3578. 2021.

Ortiga, Yasmin Y., and Romeo Luis A. Macabasag. "Temporality and Acquiescent Immobility among Aspiring Nurse Migrants in the Philippines." *Journal of Ethnic and Migration Studies* 47, no. 9 (2021): 1976–1993. https://doi.org/10.1080/1369183X.2020.1788380.

Ortiga, Yasmin Y., and Romeo Luis A. Macabasag. "Understanding International Immobility through Internal Migration: 'Left Behind' Nurses in the Philippines." *International Migration Review* 55, no. 2 (2021): 460–481. https://doi.org/10.1177/0197918320952042.

Osterman, Paul. *Who Will Care for Us? Long-Term Care and the Long-Term Workforce.* New York: Russell Sage Foundation, 2017. https://doi.org/10.7758/9781610448673.

Padios, Jan M. *A Nation on the Line: Call Centers as Postcolonial Predicaments in the Philippines.* Durham: Duke University Press, 2018.

Paligutan, P. James. *Lured by the American Dream: Filipino Servants in the US Navy and Coast Guard, 1952–1970.* Urbana: University of Illinois Press, 2022.

Parrado, Emilio A., Chris McQuiston, and Chenoa A. Flippen. "Participatory Survey Research: Integrating Community Collaboration and Quantitative Methods for the Study of Gender and HIV Risks among Hispanic Migrants." *Sociological Methods & Research* 34, no. 2 (2005): 204–239. https://doi.org/10.1177/0049124105280202.

Parreñas, Rhacel Salazar. "The Gender Paradox in the Transnational Families of Filipino Migrant Women." *Asian and Pacific Migration Journal* 14, no. 3 (2005): 243–268. https://doi.org/10.1177%2F011719680501400301.

Patel, Viraj V., Swapnil Rajpathak, and Alison Karasz. "Bangladeshi Immigrants in New York City: A Community-Based Health Needs Assessment of a Hard to Reach Population." *Journal of Immigrant and Minority Health* 14, no. 5 (2012): 767–773. https://doi.org/10.1007/s10903-011-9555-5.

Pe-Pua, Rogelia. "From Decolonizing Psychology to the Development of a Cross-Indigenous Perspective in Methodology." In *Indigenous and Cultural Psychology: Understanding People in Context*, edited by Uichol Kim, Kuo-Shu Yang, and Kwang-Kuo Hwang, 109–137. New York: Springer, 2006.

Pellow, David, and Lisa Sun-Hee Park. *The Silicon Valley of Dreams: Environmental Injustice, Immigrant Workers, and the High-Tech Global Economy.* New York: NYU Press, 2002.

Perillo, J. Lorenzo. *Choreographing in Color: Filipinos, Hip-Hop, and the Cultural Politics of Euphemism.* New York: Oxford University Press, 2020.

Perrea, Juan F. "The Echoes of Slavery: Recognizing the Racist Origins of the Agricultural and Domestic Worker Exclusion from the National Labor Relations Act." 72 *Ohio State Law Journal* 95 (2011).

Pido, Eric J. *Migrant Returns: Manila, Development, and Transnational Connectivity.* Durham: Duke University Press, 2017.

Piepzna-Samarasinha, Leah Lakshmi. *Care Work: Dreaming Disability Justice.* Vancouver: Arsenal Pulp Press, 2018.

Pilkonis, Paul A., Seung W. Choi, Steven P. Reise, Angela M. Stover, William T. Riley, David Cella, and PROMIS Cooperative Group. "Item Banks for Measuring Emotional Distress from the Patient-Reported Outcomes Measurement Information System (PROMIS®): Depression, Anxiety, and Anger." *Assessment* 18, no. 3 (2011): 263–283. https://doi.org/10.1177/1073191111411667.

Pitti, Stephen J. *The Devil in Silicon Valley: Northern California, Race, and Mexican Americans.* Princeton: Princeton University Press, 2002.

Portes, Alejandro, and Min Zhou. "The New Second Generation: Segmented Assimilation and Its Variants." *Annals of the American Academy of Political and Social Science* 530, no. 1 (1993): 74–96. https://doi.org/10.1177/0002716293530001006.

Reid, Alison, Elena Ronda-Perez, and Marc B. Schenker. "Migrant Workers, Essential Work, and COVID-19." *American Journal of Industrial Medicine* 64, no. 2 (2021): 73–77. https://doi.org/10.1002/ajim.23209.

Reyes, Victoria. "Ethnographic Toolkit: Strategic Positionality and Researchers' Visible and Invisible Tools in Field Research." *Ethnography* 21, no. 2 (2020): 220–240. https://doi.org/10.1177/1466138118805121.

Riley, Kevin, Jennifer Nazareno, and Sterling Malish. "24-Hour Care: Work and Sleep Conditions of Migrant Filipino Live-In Caregivers in Los Angeles." *American Journal of Industrial Medicine* 59, no. 12 (2016): 1120–1129. https://doi.org/10.1002/ajim.22647.

Roberts, J. Timmons. "Psychosocial Effects of Workplace Hazardous Exposures: Theoretical Synthesis and Preliminary Findings." *Social Problems* 40, no. 1 (1993): 74–89. https://doi.org/10.2307/3097027.

Robinson, Cedric J. *Black Marxism: The Making of the Black Radical Tradition.* Revised and updated 3rd edition. Chapel Hill: University of North Carolina Press, 2020.

Rodriguez, Robyn M. *Filipino American Transnational Activism: Diasporic Politics among the Second Generation.* Vol. 1. Leiden, The Netherlands: Brill, 2019.

Rodriguez, Robyn Magalit. *Migrants for Export: How the Philippine State Brokers Labor to the World.* Minneapolis: University of Minnesota Press, 2010.

Ruiz, Neil G. "Made for Export: Labor Migration, State Power, and Higher Education in a Developing Philippine Economy." PhD diss. Massachusetts Institute of Technology, 2014.

Rumbaut, Ruben G. "Ages, Life Stages, and Generational Cohorts: Decomposing the Immigrant First and Second Generations in the United States." *International Migration Review* 38, no. 3 (2004): 1160–1205. https://doi.org/10.1111%2Fj.1747-7379.2004.tb00232.x.

Sabon, Lauren Copley. "Force, Fraud, and Coercion—What Do They Mean? A Study of Victimization Experiences in a New Destination Latino Sex Trafficking Network." *Feminist Criminology* 13, no. 5 (2018): 456-476.

Saguin, Kidjie. "Returning Broke and Broken? Return Migration, Reintegration, and Transnational Social Protection in the Philippines." *Migration and Development* 9, no. 3 (2020): 352-368. https://doi.org/10.1080/21632324.2020.1787100.

Sales, Joy. "Martial Law Histories from a Critical Filipina/x/o American Perspective." *Amerasia Journal* 48, no. 1 (2022): 91-93. https://doi.org/10.1080/00447471.2022.2152270.

Sales, Joy N. "#NeverAgainToMartialLaw: Transnational Filipino American Activism in the Shadow of Marcos and Age of Duterte." *Amerasia Journal* 45, no. 3 (2019): 299-315. https://doi.org/10.1080/00447471.2019.1715702.

Sanchez, Mark John. "Let the People Speak: Solidarity Culture and the Making of a Transnational Opposition to the Marcos Dictatorship, 1972-1986." PhD diss. University of Illinois, 2018.

Sangalang, Cindy C. "'I'm Sick of Being Called a Hero—I Want to Get Paid Like One': Filipino American Frontline Workers' Health under Conditions of COVID-19 and Racial Capitalism." *Frontiers in Public Health* 10 (November 2022): 977-955. https://doi.org/10.3389/fpubh.2022.977955.

Schulze-Oechtering, Michael. "'Anti-Marcos Filipinos' and Other Anti-Imperialist Diasporas: The Solidarity Politics of the Committee for Justice for Domingo and Viernes's (CJDV)." *Alon: Journal for Filipinx American and Diasporic Studies* 1, no. 1 (2021). https://doi.org/10.5070/LN41149592.

Shah, Hina B. "Understaffed and Overworked: Poor Working Conditions and Quality of Care in Residential Care Facilities for the Elderly." *Publications* (May 2017): 788.

Siu, Lok, and Claire Chun. "Yellow Peril and Techno-Orientalism in the Time of Covid-19: Racialized Contagion, Scientific Espionage, and Techno-Economic Warfare." *Journal of Asian American Studies* 23, no. 3 (2020): 421-440.

Smith, Linda Tuhiwai. *Decolonizing Methodologies: Research and Indigenous Peoples.* London: Zed Books, 1999.

Smith, Ted, and Phil Woodward. *The Legacy of High Tech Development: The Toxic Lifecycle of Computer Manufacturing.* San Jose, CA: Silicon Valley Toxics Coalition, 1992.

Soehl, Thomas, and Roger Waldinger. "Inheriting the Homeland? Intergenerational Transmission of Cross-Border Ties in Migrant Families." *American Journal of Sociology* 118, no. 3 (2012): 778-813. https://doi.org/10.1086/667720.

Suzuki, Ayame. "The Philippines' Response to COVID-19: Limits of State Capacity." *Corona Chronicles: Voices from the Field* (blog), June 29, 2020. https://covid-19chronicles.cseas.kyoto-u.ac.jp/post-046-html.

Tabb, William K. *The Amoral Elephant: Globalization and the Struggle for Social Justice in the Twenty-First Century.* New York: Monthly Review Press, 2001.

Tadiar, Neferti Xina Maca. *Fantasy Production: Sexual Economies and Other Philippine Consequences for the New World Order*. Hong Kong: Hong Kong University Press, 2004.

Tamanal, Jerre Mae, Kyung Eun Park, and Cheong Hoon Kim. "The Relationship of Perceived Stress and Lifestyle Choices among Filipino Adolescents." *International Research Journal of Public and Environmental Health* 4, no. 10 (2017): 205–214. https://doi.org/10.15739/irjpeh.17.025.

Teehankee, Julio C. "Duterte's Pandemic Populism." *United Nations University World Institute for Development Economics Research*, 2022. https://www.wider.unu.edu/publication/duterte%E2%80%99s-pandemic-populism.

Tessler, Hannah, Meera Choi, and Grace Kao. "The Anxiety of Being Asian American: Hate Crimes and Negative Biases during the COVID-19 Pandemic." *American Journal of Criminal Justice* 45 (2020): 636-646.

Thompson, Maddy. "The Philippines' Business Process Outsourcing Industry through COVID-19." *LSE Southeast Asia* (blog) (2022). https://blogs.lse.ac.uk/seac/2020/09/22/covid-19-and-the-philippines-outsourcing-industry.

Tintiangco-Cubales, Allyson, Rita Kohli, Jocyl Sacramento, Nick Henning, Ruchi Agarwal-Rangnath, and Christine Sleeter. "Toward an Ethnic Studies Pedagogy: Implications for K-12 Schools from the Research." *Urban Review* 47 (2015): 104–125. https://doi.org/10.1007/s11256-014-0280-y.

Tintiangco-Cubales, Allyson, and Jocyl Sacramento. "Practicing Pinayist Pedagogy." *Amerasia Journal* 35, no. 1 (2009): 179–187. https://doi.org/10.17953/amer.35.1.98257024r4501756.

Tiongson, Antonio T. "On Rethinking the Politics and Possibilities of Joy." *Alon: Journal for Filipinx American and Diasporic Studies* 2, no. 2 (2022): 169–171. https://www.jstor.org/stable/48680004.

Todd, Anne Marie. *Valley of Heart's Delight: Environment and Sense of Place in the Santa Clara Valley*. Berkeley: University of California Press, 2022.

Torre, Maria, and Michelle Fine. "Participatory Action Research (PAR) by Youth." In *Youth Activism: An International Encyclopedia*, edited by Lonnie R. Sherrod, Constance A. Flanagan, Ron Kassimir, and Amy K. Syvertsen, 456–462. Westport, CT: Greenwood, 2006.

Tronto, Joan C. "Creating Caring Institutions: Politics, Plurality, and Purpose." *Ethics and Social Welfare* 4, no. 2 (2010): 158–171. https://doi.org/10.1080/17496535.2010.484259.

Tsu, Cecilia M. *Garden of the World: Asian Immigrants and the Making of Agriculture in California's Santa Clara Valley*. New York: Oxford University Press, 2013.

Tuck, Eve. "Re-Visioning Action: Participatory Action Research and Indigenous Theories of Change." *Urban Review* 41 (September 2008): 47–65. https://doi.org/10.1007/s11256-008-0094-x.

Tung, Charlene. "The Cost of Caring: The Social Reproductive Labor of Filipina Live-in Home Health Caregivers." *Frontiers: A Journal of Women Studies* 21, nos. 1/2 (2000): 61–82. https://doi.org/10.2307/3347032.

Tungohan, Ethel. *Care Activism: Migrant Domestic Workers, Movement-Building, and Communities of Care*. Urbana: University of Illinois Press, 2023.

———. "Reconceptualizing Motherhood, Reconceptualizing Resistance: Migrant Domestic Workers, Transnational Hyper-Maternalism, and Activism." *International Feminist Journal of Politics* 15, no. 1 (2013): 39–57. https://doi.org/10.1080/14616742.2012.699781.

Tyner, James A. *The Philippines: Mobilities, Identities, Globalization*. New York: Taylor & Francis US, 2009.

Ullah, A. K. M. Ahsan, Faraha Nawaz, and Diotima Chattoraj. "Locked Up under Lockdown: The COVID-19 Pandemic and the Migrant Population." *Social Sciences & Humanities Open* 3, no. 1 (2021): 100–126. https://doi.org/10.1016/j.ssaho.2021.100126.

Unger, Hella von. "Participatory Health Research with Immigrant Communities in Germany." *International Journal of Action Research* 8, no. 3 (2012): 266–287. https://doi.org/10.1688/1861-9916_IJAR_2012_03_Unger.

Uy-Tioco, Cecilia S., and Earvin Charles B. Cabalquinto. "Transnational Mobile Carework: Filipino Migrants, Family Intimacy, and Mobile Media." In *Mobile Media and Social Intimacies in Asia*, edited by Jason Vincent A. Cabañales and Cecilia S. Uy-Tioco, 153–170. New York City: Palgrave Macmillan, 2020.

van der Velde, Jeannette, Deanna L. Williamson, and Linda D. Ogilvie. "Participatory Action Research: Practical Strategies for Actively Engaging and Maintaining Participation in Immigrant and Refugee Communities." *Qualitative Health Research* 19, no. 9 (2009): 1293–1302. https://doi.org/10.1177/1049732309344207.

Velasco, Gina K. *Queering the Global Filipina Body: Contested Nationalisms in the Filipina/o Diaspora*. Urbana: University of Illinois Press, 2020.

Vergara, Benito Manalo. *Pinoy Capital: The Filipino Nation in Daly City*. Philadelphia: Temple University Press, 2009.

Verret, April. "How Racist Policies Continue to Hurt Home Care Workers." *Time* (2020). https://time.com/5882416/home-care-workers-racism.

Villegas, Mark R. *Manifest Technique: Hip Hop, Empire, and Visionary Filipino American Culture*. Vol. 1. Urbana: University of Illinois Press, 2021.

Vilog, Ron Bridget T., and Carlos M. Piocos III. "Community of Care amid Pandemic Inequality: The Case of Filipino Migrant Domestic Workers in the UK, Italy, and Hong Kong." *Asia-Pacific Social Science Review* 21, no. 2 (2021): 184–201.

Viola, Michael Joseph. "Toward a Filipino/a Critical (FilCrit) Pedagogy: A Study of United States Educational Exposure Programs to the Philippines." PhD diss. University of California, Los Angeles, 2012.

Vizheh, Maryam, Mostafa Qorbani, Seyed Masoud Arzaghi, Salut Muhidin, Zohreh Javanmard, and Marzieh Esmaeili. "The Mental Health of Healthcare Workers in the COVID-19 Pandemic: A Systematic Review." *Journal of Diabetes & Metabolic Disorders* 19, no. 2 (2020): 1967–1978. https://doi.org/10.1007/s40200-020-00643-9.

Watson, Tony J. 2008. *Sociology, Work and Industry*. New York: Routledge.

Williams, Sharon Wallace, and Peggye Dilworth-Anderson. "Systems of Social Support in Families Who Care for Dependent African American Elders." *The Gerontologist* 42, no. 2 (2002): 224–236. https://doi.org/10.1093/geront/42.2.224.

Wong, Tiffany. "Little Noticed, Filipino Americans Are Dying of COVID-19 at an Alarming Rate." *Los Angeles Times*, July 21, 2020. https://www.latimes.com/california/story/2020-07-21/filipino-americans-dying-covid.

Woodly, Deva, Rachel H. Brown, Mara Marin, Shatema Threadcraft, Christopher Paul Harris, Jasmine Syedullah, and Miriam Ticktin. "The Politics of Care." *Contemporary Political Theory* 20, no. 4 (2021): 890–925.

Yeoh, Brenda S. A., and Shirlena Huang. 2000. "'Home' and 'Away': Foreign Domestic Workers and Negotiations of Diasporic Identity in Singapore." *Women's Studies International Forum* 23, no. 4: 413–429. https://doi.org/10.1016/S0277-5395(00)00105-9.

Yeoh, Brenda S. A., Katie D. Willis, and S. M. Abdul Khader Fakhri. "Introduction: Transnationalism and Its Edges." *Ethnic and Racial Studies* 26, no. 2 (2003): 207–217. https://doi.org/10.1080/0141987032000054394.

Yeung, C. Y., Bishan Huang Nelson, Christine Y. K. Lau, and Joseph T. F. Lau. "Feeling Anxious amid the COVID-19 Pandemic: Psychosocial Correlates of Anxiety Symptoms among Filipina Domestic Helpers in Hong Kong." *International Journal of Environmental Research and Public Health* 17, no. 21 (2020): 8102. https://doi.org/10.3390/ijerph17218102.

Yoo, Grace J., and Barbara W. Kim. *Caring across Generations: The Linked Lives of Korean American Families*. New York: NYU Press, 2014.

INDEX

The letter *f* following a page number denotes a figure.

abuse: emotional 8, 76; physical, 93; verbal, 8, 76
acute care, 19, 60, 153–154. *See also* nonmedical care workers
agencies: city, 99; employment, 7–9, 46, 65–66, 72–76, 150; for-profit, 7; mental health, 156; private, 19; recruitment, 14, 96–97; state departments, 20, 112, 129, 150. *See also* Overseas Workers Welfare Agency; Philippine Overseas Employment Agency
Alice: caregiving, 95; recruitment, 95; trafficking, 97; work experience, 96
Alicia: caregiving, 58; daily risks due to pandemic, 60
Alma: caregiving, 40
Americans with Disabilities Act, 15
amnesty, 148
anchor migrant, 10
anti-Asian racism: pandemic, 61, 74; President Trump's remarks, 72–73; scarce work opportunities, 76–77
anxiety: and depression, 44; Justine, 69; Miriam, 93; pandemic, 26, 59, 68, 100, 156

assisted living facility, 18–19, 60, 62, 101
assisted residential facility, 8, 19, 70; live-in caregivers, 51; oversight by state agencies, 20; privatized, 46; variation among programs, 20; work conditions for caregivers, 25

Baby Boomer generation, 6
Banta, Vanessa, 69
bayanihan, 116–118
BAYAN Philippines, 126
Bay Area: and anchor ethnic enclave, 11; chain migration, 1–2, 10; "communities of care", 88; family petitions, 12; Filipino caregivers, 46, 96, 103; grassroots organizations, xi, 106, 109, 156; Hart-Cellar Act of 1965, 9; horticulture industry history, 9–10; kuwentuhan, 130; larger Filipino community, 15, 80, 135; PAWIS, x, 119; setting for data collection, 22–23, 61, 122, 125, 132, 134; vulnerability of caregivers, 19, 62, 154. *See also* Daly City, CA; Silicon Valley
Boston, MA, 82

195

breaks: California Domestic Workers Bill breaks of Rights, 47; coffee, 108; cut short, 20, 44, 46–48; meal, 12, 22, 44, 46, 48; workday, 41, 48, 64. *See also* kapihan
Brenner, Johanna, 35
Brillante, Tess, 134

Cahill, Caitlin, 145
California Department of Social Services and Community Care Licensing, 20
California Domestic Workers Bill of Rights, 47, 159
California Domestic Workers Coalition (CDWC), 159–160
California Occupational Safety and Health Act (Cal/OSHA), 82, 160
call centers, 78
capitalism: global, 15; and labor process for caregivers, 17–18; late-stage, 113, 147; racial, 4, 13, 91, 98, 147, 152. *See also* social reproductive labor
"caregivers' contradiction," 25, 37, 45
caregivers' health and wellness: Cal/OSHA, 160; fears about, 59; limited labor protections, 82, 87, 151; mental, 52; physical, 43, 52, 69; research about, 134. *See also* "caregivers' contradiction"
CARE Project: background, 21, 136, 143, 157; kuwentuhan sessions, 116–119, 156; as political education, 132
care work, 5, 8, 34; marketization of a public good, 92, 94, 112; racialized and gendered history of exploitation, 18, 152; transactional definition, 92–93; unpaid, 17, 90. *See also* devaluation of care work; "Filipino work ethic"; social reproductive labor

Carlos, Edwin, xii, 130
Carmela: anxiety, 100; shared housing, 99, 101
CDWC (California Domestic Workers Coalition), 159–160
Cebu City, 150
Celemen, Elaika, xii; CARE Project, 136; kuwentuhan sessions, 23; survey research, 134
certified nurse assistant (CNA), 6, 18, 62, 80
chain migration, 2, 10
Charylle: working through pain, 43
Che: residential care facility, 48
Cherry: residential care facility, 79
CNA (certified nurse assistant), 6, 18, 62, 80
Colen, Shellee, 14, 17, 112. *See also* stratified reproduction
communication technologies, 77, 108, 112. *See also specific technologies*
"communities of care", 27, 88; *The Labor of Care*, 26; social reproductive labor, 89, 91; theorizing about, 91, 101, 110–111, 113, 145
companions, 12, 14, 131
consumer, 7, 12; caregiving for elders, 25, 46, 50; lack of understanding, 71; risks for, 21, 50
contracts, 7, 151; coercive nature of, 97
COVID-19: changing information about, 21, 50, 67, 70, 121; contraction, 19, 59, 61, 67, 75; death, 19, 61, 79, 82, 154; failure of privatized care, 18–19; testing, 24, 80, 150. *See also* anti-Asian racism; pandemic; PPE
cultural traits, 14
"culture-centered approach," 45, 132
Cynthia: working through pain, 78

196 / INDEX

Daly City, CA: chain migration, 9–10
de Borja, Jean Aaron, 76, 90, 102
debt: bondage, 96; filial, 53–54; to recruitment agencies, 1, 14. *See also* utang ng loob
depression, 44, 52, 71, 156. *See also* anxiety
devaluation of care work, 13, 16, 60, 81, 92. *See also* "normalized exploitation"
Diana: detailed daily schedule, 47–48; residential care facility, 47
Dilworth-Anderson, Peggye, 34
direct care worker, 6, 18, 20
"disposable" people, 4, 15–16, 46, 60, 154
"doing family," 79

eldercare: caregivers made invisible, 60, 88, 151; and caregivers' race and gender, 34; crisis of, 25, 45, 86, 154; political power and organizing of migrant workers, 16, 160; poorly funded systems, 13, 101, 152–153; privatization of, 8, 11, 16, 20, 23, 46
Ellen: daily risks due to pandemic, 60, 80
employment agencies, 46, 72, 76
employment arrangements, 7–8, 20, 46

Facebook, 77, 79, 108
FaceTime, 77, 79, 108
Fair Labor Standards Act (FLSA): racialized and gendered legacy, 72; violating tenets of, 12, 81–82
FAJ (Filipinos Advocating for Justice), 109–110
Felicia: anti-Asian racism, 73
Filipino Community Center, 21, 115–116, 118, 133f; Workers' Rights Program, 131. *See also* PAR
Filipinos Advocating for Justice (FAJ), 109–110

"Filipino work ethic," 32, 37, 45. *See also* "no work, no pay"
FLSA (Fair Labor Standards Act). *See* Fair Labor Standards Act
formal care worker, 6
Francisco, Remedios Luna, 28f, 29, 147–148; daily schedule, 30–33, 47–48

GABRIELA, 116, 126
GABRIELA NYC, 131
GABRIELA San Francisco, 21, 116, 131, 133f
gamble of labor migration, 90, 151
Gilmore, Ruthie Wilson, 15, 164n42
Grace: anti-Asian racism, 73–74
Guevarra, Anna Romina: "labor brokerage state," 14
Gutierrez, Armand, 139

health insurance: employment agencies, 7; lack of, 22, 37–38, 40, 75
Hester: lack of health insurance, 37
Hobart, Hi'ilei, 91
housekeepers, 14, 103, 159

Ian: residential care facility, 62
Immigration Act (1965), 10
increased workloads, 151
informal immigrant networks, 46, 65: churches, 125; community organizations, 26, 65, 91, 144, 157, 160
information and communication technologies (ICTs), 77, 108, 112. *See also specific technologies*
In-Home Support Services, 7
insider, 2
Instagram, 77, 108
intergenerational dialogue, 25, 122, 157; filial obligation to parents, 138–139. *See also* kuwentuhan

INDEX / *197*

interruptions: breaks, 47; meal, 12; rest, 12; sleep, 12, 20, 47
intragenerational dialogue, 138, 141, 144
"invisible front line," 61, 70–71
Irma: fear and panic at the onset of pandemic, 68; risks of caregiving, 69
Isaac, Allan Punzalan: caregivers' innovative practices, 112–113; Filipino Time, 91
isolation: caregivers in the workplace, 8, 26, 68, 96, 107; pandemic protocols, 24, 156, 158

Jenni: preexisting health conditions, 72
Jess: family work history, 11
Josie: daily risks due to pandemic, 58–60
Justine: anxiety, 69; personal health, 70; stress, 69

kababayan, 86, 90, 94, 110
Kalinga, Philippines, 127
kamustahan, 57
Kang, Miliann, 74
kapihan, 108
kapwa, 97–98, 110, 125, 129
Kneese, Tamara, 91
Kristal: kuwentuhan session, 155–156
Kristine: risks as a caregiver, 78
kuwento, 49, 118, 129, 145
kuwentuhan: critical Filipinx American studies collective, 133f, 144–146; fostering trust, 110, 129; intergenerational understanding, 137–139; method, 24, 118–119, 121, 132; praxis, 124–125; research training, 118, 134; source of knowledge, 22–23, 130–131; virtual format, 120, 135–136, 158–159. *See also* pakikipagkuwentuhan

labor exploitation, 8, 125
Laslett, Barbara, 35
Laura: daily work schedule 49; residential care facility, 49–50
Leif: remittances, 41–42
Lia: lack of access to part-time work, 66
Linda: lack of access to part-time work, 41, 66; mental health, 70; verbal abuse, 70–71
long-term care: caregiver testimonials, 69; "formal care workers," 6; hot spots for COVID-19 transmission, 86; immigration to the US, 1, 4; lack of protections and information about COVID-19, 19–20, 60, 67, 88, 147; larger healthcare chain, 16, 70, 151–152; neoliberal governance of, 8, 76, 87, 94, 153. *See also* residential care facilities
Lorraine: intensified work during pandemic, 63–64
Los Angeles, CA, 11

Mabalon, Dawn Bohulano, 123
Manila: port city, 150; recruitment of workers to the US, 112; Spanish Manila Galleon Trades, 123; transnational ties, 39
Marcos, Ferdinand, 122
Mari: remittances, 79; risks as a caregiver, 78
Marxist feminist, 16–17, 89. *See also* class analysis
Medicaid, 7–8, 16, 18
Medicare, 8, 16
Michelle: risks as a caregiver, 39
MIGRANTE NYC, 131
Miriam: pain of loss, 102; physical abuse, 93
Mondina, Felwina, 134

Nadasen, Premilla, 8
Nanet: anxiety, 100; shared housing, 99, 101
nannies, 14, 103, 158; mobilizing and organizing, 159. *See also* labor brokerage state; social reproductive labor
Nasol, Katherine, 4, 20–21, 49, 86, 98, 152
Nazareno, Jennifer, 94
neoliberal: crisis in caregiving, 26, 83; divestment in social welfare, 46, 92; governance of care, 4, 152; Philippines' relationship to other nations, 150; radical care and mutual aid, 91, 111; sending states, 112; US health care, 18, 21, 76, 98
New York City: research conducted, 125–126, 129, 131; workers' transnational ties to the Philippines, 79, 88
Nishida, Akemi, 18
nonmedical: care workers, 19; facilities, 12, 19. *See also* acute care
"normalized exploitation," 45–46, 50, 92. *See also* devaluation of care work
"no work, no pay": "caregivers' contradiction," 25; guiding philosophy, 39, 42; informal networks of resource sharing, 51; kuwentuhan sessions, 36–37; work ethic, 45, 55. *See also* Filipino work ethic
nurses: deaths from COVID-19, 18, 80, 154; Filipino, 4, 7, 12, 18, 80, 154; licensed vocational, 80; research about, 94; risks during pandemic, 67, 152, 155; trafficking, 97. *See also* CNAs; Nazareno, Jennifer
nursing homes: hot spots for COVID-19 transmission, 86; lack of protections and funding for workers, 19–20; privatized, 8

Occupational Safety and Health Act, California (Cal/OSHA), 82, 160
Osorio, Kristal, xii; CARE Project, 136; kuwentuhan sessions, 23; survey research, 134
Overseas Filipino Worker (OFW), 151
Overseas Workers Welfare Agency, 150
overtime pay protections, 12

pain of loss, 102
pakikipagkuwentuhan: talk-story, 129, 143. *See also* storytelling
pakikipagsapalaran, 99, 104; Jean de Borja, 90, 102, 104; Neferti Tadiar, 90, 101–102
pandemic: lockdown period, 21, 50, 57, 73, 87, 108; shifts in work and wages, 63–64; shut down communication between employers and caregivers, 20, 158. *See also* COVID-19
PAR. *See* participatory action research
paradox of essential workers, 59
Parreñas Shimizu, Celine, 146
participatory action research (PAR): kuwentuhan, 139, 142; local political organizing, 126–128, 131–134, 145; methodology, 21–22, 25, 126, 129–130; *Migration Letters*, 128; transnational analysis, 137–139
part-time work, 8, 63, 65–67. *See also* informal immigrant networks
PAWIS (Pilipino Association of Workers and Immigrants), 109–110, 145f; filing wage theft cases, 85; kuwentuhan sessions, 39–40, 51, 57, 68, 120, 134; PPE drop-offs, 153; worker leaders, 86, 105–106, 108. *See also* Teresa; Tita Megan
personal care assistant, 6

personal care attendant, 6
personal protective equipment (PPE), 19–21, 26, 51, 58; caregivers sharing information about resources, 99–100, 113, 134, 144; not given out by employers, 64
Philippine Overseas Employment Agency, 150
physical exhaustion, 44
Piepzna-Samarasinha, Leah Lakshmi, 122
Pilipino Association of Workers and Immigrants. *See* PAWIS
Pinky: working through pain, 40
port cities, 11, 150. *See also* Los Angeles, CA; Manila, Philippines; San Francisco, CA
PPE. *See* personal protective equipment
Pratt, Geraldine, 69
privatization: of eldercare, 8, 11, 13, 20, 92
public transportation, 67, 71
Puri, 3, 43, 54

racism and discrimination: systemic, 72, 80
radical care, 21, 27, 89, 91, 113, 122–124
Rae, 40
recipient, 7, 14, 18, 139
relationality, 91, 102
remittances, 36, 40, 52, 54; and communal living arrangements, 101; Philippines' national reliance, 78–79; sacrifices and later generations, 124, 139. *See also* utang ng loob
repatriation, 78, 151
residential care facilities, 8, 12, 19, 29, 70; Che, 48; Cherry, 79; Diana, 47; devaluation of care workers, 60, 70; Filipino owners of, 13; health and safety risks to caregivers, 18, 53, 82; Ian, 62; Laura, 49–50; live-in caregivers, 51; Michelle, 39; oversight by state agencies, 20; privatized, 46; Rowena, 63; variation among programs, 20; violating tenets of FLSA, 12, 81–82; work conditions for caregivers, 25
responsibility: community of caregivers, 21; gendered, 35; privatized health care, 8, 26; training for caregivers, 6, 8; transnational ties to families in the Philippines, 25, 34–38, 41–43, 52, 81
retaliation: fear or threat of, 12, 107; from employers, 8, 20
Rica, 94
Richelle: distance from family in the Philippines, 53–54; support with other caregivers, 103–104; *tiis*, 103; utang ng loob, 54; working through pain, 38
Rina: activism with FAJ, 109–110; caregiving, 95; debt peonage and recruitment agency, 96; risk and protection in the pandemic, 67; trafficking, 97
Roanna: anti-Asian racism, 73
Rodriguez, Robyn: CARE Project, 21; "Filipinx Count!" survey, 24; "labor brokerage state," 14, 122; PAR, 131, 134
Rosselle: diabetes, 67; risks to personal health, 67–68
Rowena: residential care facility, 63
Rumbaut, Ruben, 123

salamat circle of community, 118, 119f. *See also* pagsasalamat
San Francisco, CA: caregiver activism and research, 22–23, 119, 121–122, 130; ethnic labor niche, 46; Filipino Community Center, x, 115; immigration history, 9–11; municipal response to COVID-19 pandemic, 19–20. *See also* Bay Area

San Francisco State University, 21, 22, 136; CARE Project, 132; League of Filipino Students, 116; Pilipino American Collegiate Endeavor, xi

Santa Clara County Department of Public Health, 87f

Serena: remittances, 52; stress, 52; tiis, 53; working through pain, 42–43

Sheila: anti-Asian racism, 76; risk and protection in the pandemic, 51; tiis, 33

Sherry, 71

Silicon Valley: caregivers, 85, 99; history, 10; PAWIS, 57, 105, 108, 134; technology industries, 9, 11

social reproductive labor, 15, 91; Shellee Colen, 14; Marxist feminist scholars, 16–17, 35, 89, 147; "neoliberal governance of care," 4; sudden loss of work, 159

storytelling, 22, 124, 143. *See also* kuwentuhan; pakikipagkuwentuhan

stratified reproduction, 14, 17, 112

stress: CARE Project, 132; "culture-centered approach," 45; Filipino caregivers, 3, 22–23, 52, 69; indicators, 44; nakakastress, 66; pakikipagkuwentuhan, 143; research about, 82; workplace, 53

stressors, 26, 55, 67, 105, 152; mental health, 52–53, 68, 150, 152

Sudafed, 75

Susanna, 59

Sylvia, 100; shared housing, 99, 101

Tadiar, Neferti: Fantasy Production, 90–91

Taggueg, R. J., 24, 134, 136

taxes and deductions, 7. *See also* agencies

technology industry, 9, 11. *See also* Silicon Valley

Teresa: activism as worker leader with PAWIS, 86–89, 105–106, 113; filing wage theft case, 85; kababayan, 90; stress, 86; trafficking, 97. *See also* "communities of care"

tiis (resolve), 55, 98; Richelle, 103; Serena, 53; Sheila, 33

Tita Megan, 58. *See also* PAWIS

Tracy: lack of health insurance, 75

Trump, Donald, 72. *See also* anti-Asian racism

Tungohan, Ethel, xiv, 110

Typhoon Haiyan, 140

Uber, 58, 71, 155

uncertain work conditions, 59, 61, 77, 80, 91–92, 151; fear of, 62, 81

undocumented workers: filing for "amnesty," 148; job losses during pandemic, 20, 104; lack of protections for caregivers, 18, 60, 97; nakakagaan ng loob, 105

University of California, Berkeley, 136

University of California, Davis, 136; Bulosan Center for Filipinx Studies, xii, 24, 134; Robyn Rodriguez, 131

University of San Francisco, 21, 131

utang ng loob: caregivers and, 54–55, 95; as social reciprocity, 23, 53, 98

Viber, 77

visas: "anchor migrant," 10; chain migration, 12; expiring, 2, 150; temporary, 96–97

wage: anxiety around, 100; filing wage theft case, 85, 105; hourly, 8, 65, 67; low,

wage (*continued*)
    93, 96, 98, 101, 109, 112, 134; minimum, 81; part-time, 110; and privatization, 92; theft, 85–86, 106, 120–121, 131–133; violating FLSA, 82

WhatsApp, 51, 77, 108

Williams, Sharon Wallace, 34

word of mouth, 7, 12, 153

worker benefits, 7, 21, 67, 72, 108, 152

workers' compensation, 7, 16, 36, 40

working through pain/poor health, 37–38, 40, 42–43, 93; back, 54–55, 82. *See also* abuse

"yellow peril" discourse, 72

Zoom, 19, 113; interviews, 73, 78; kapihan, 108; kuwentuhan, 24–25, 57, 109, 120, 135–136, 158–159; work and school, 107. *See also* PAWIS